SEASONS OF CARING

Meditations for Alzheimer's and Dementia Caregivers

Edited by

Dr. Daniel C. Potts, Editor-in-Chief

Lynda Everman

Rabbi Steven M. Glazer

Dr. Richard L. Morgan

Max Wallack

ClergyAgainstAlzheimer's | A Network of USAgainstAlzheimer's

ClergyAgainstAlzheimer's Network, Publisher

Seasons of Caring: Meditations for Alzheimer's and Dementia Caregivers

Copyright © ClergyAgainstAlzheimer's Network, 2014

ISBN 978-1502936134

Publication Date 12/2014

ABOUT THE ARTWORK

The artwork on the book's cover and seasonal sections was created by Lester E. Potts, Jr. while he was a client at Caring Days Adult Dementia Daycare Center (The Mal and Charlotte Moore Center) in Tuscaloosa, Alabama. A rural saw miller who had never previously shown any artistic talent, Lester became a watercolor artist in the throes of Alzheimer's disease, and his art has been displayed from Beverly Hills, California to Paris, France.

The painting displayed on the cover is a favorite of the Potts family primarily for what it says metaphorically. No longer floating in the water and of value for its traditional usefulness, the boat has been cast aside and abandoned on the shore. But grace and life draw forth beauty from the wreckage. This is what Lester experienced, and what can happen to many others with dementia and their caregivers, as well.

DEDICATION

To those with Alzheimer's and dementia and all who love them.

CONTENTS

SUMMER

TRANSITIONS

FALL

WINTER

ARTWORK *by Lester E. Potts, Jr. (with descriptions by Daniel C. Potts)*

FOREWORD

Our mission at USAgainstAlzheimer's is to stop this disease by 2020. Alzheimer's and dementia affect over five million Americans and their families and 44 million people worldwide. Mine was one of those families. My mom was a scrappy, heroic, lioness of a woman. She was invincible—or so I thought—but she was no match for Alzheimer's. Every day since she lost her battle to this unforgiving disease, I miss her. And every day, I try to summon her grit in our battle to stop Alzheimer's.

My husband, George, and I started USAgainstAlzheimer's to spare other families from this cruel disease—the only leading cause of death still on the rise. Every doctor and scientist fighting Alzheimer's on the front lines tells us the same thing: If we want to prevent, treat or cure Alzheimer's by 2020, we need more research funding. So we raise our voices in Congress and the White House demanding more money for research. We break down barriers by bringing scientists and industry together. We work with global leaders to speed up discovery of new Alzheimer's therapies. And we work with caregivers who join us and help bring Alzheimer's and dementia out of the shadows.

We also support families who are living with Alzheimer's. Our ClergyAgainstAlzheimer's Network harnesses the powerful voices of men and women of faith to call for urgent action to stop this disease, and for better, more compassionate care for those with Alzheimer's and their families. To this end, the Clergy Network has created *Seasons of Caring*, a first-of-its-kind interfaith volume that speaks to the unique challenges faced by Alzheimer's and dementia caregivers. You'll find original and beautiful meditations by clergy and leaders from many faith traditions that offer encouragement, empathy and understanding.

I hope that *Seasons of Caring* brings you comfort, inspiration and spiritual growth during a deeply challenging time. We are confronted with the reality of Alzheimer's and dementia. What are we going to do about it? Fight for a cure and join together to care.

Trish Vradenburg
Co-Founder, USAgainstAlzheimer's

PREFACE

"To all of you, I repeat: Do not let yourselves be robbed of hope! Do not let yourselves be robbed of hope! And not only that, but I say to us all: let us not rob others of hope, let us become bearers of hope!" - Pope Francis

God's omnipotent hand truly works in many wondrous ways. It is my deepest belief that both the ClergyAgainstAlzheimer's Network and this book are products of God's hand. They are both the result of the following loosely connected series of events.

Strange as it may seem, I was away from organized religion for more than 40 years. It was late in 2009 that a neighbor invited me to attend Sunday services with her. I had just reluctantly and painfully moved my husband to an assisted living facility.

A few months later, in early 2010, George and Trish Vradenburg launched USAgainstAlzheimer's. I was immediately drawn to their bold vision of stopping Alzheimer's by 2020. Through its networks, USAgainstAlzheimer's mobilizes deeply affected communities, including women, African Americans, Latinos, researchers and caregivers. Recognizing that we are the "us" in USAgainstAlzheimer's, I quickly joined them as a founding member of both the Activists and Women's Networks. I came to believe that a network of interfaith clergy would offer an important and powerful perspective in our collective efforts to fight this disease.

With the full support of the Vradenburgs, USAgainstAlzheimer's Director Ginny Biggar and I set out to create ClergyAgainstAlzheimer's. Our efforts were accelerated when Boston University senior and neuroscience major Max Wallack volunteered to help identify faith leaders who might be interested in our cause, and when Rabbi Steven M. Glazer and Rev. Dr. Richard L. Morgan answered our call and took up the mantle to offer advice and recruit other founders. We then asked noted neurologist and author Dr. Daniel C. Potts to serve as medical advisor to our founders and to take the voice of the faith community back to his colleagues in the medical community. Our team was in place.

Initially, we had hoped to find about twenty interested clergy to be founders of this new network. Today we have over 100 founding members and are now recruiting clergy, laity and faith organizations. And in your hands is what we believe to be the first-of-its-kind, an interfaith book of meditations written by members of our network.

It was Dr. Potts who suggested the idea for a book of meditations with these words, "Here is something to think about…" Literally, overnight, our thoughts melded into this project with an outline, a book title, and a strategy for implementation. We are grateful to our authors, caregivers themselves, who so generously have given of their time, experience and counsel.

The words of Pope Francis bear repeating as they well describe the intent of Clergy AgainstAlzheimer's and *Seasons of Caring*, "Do not let yourselves be robbed of hope! And not only that…let us become bearers of hope!" Please join us! Visit www.SeasonsofCaring.org to learn more about our mission and work, as well as to find resources for faith communities, including sermons, books, programs, and actions you can take that will help us stop Alzheimer's. To all the caregivers and advocates, you are the silver lining of this insidious disease; thank you for your tireless work on behalf of others. May God provide comfort to those who suffer and move us closer to a cure.

Lynda Everman
Convener, ClergyAgainstAlzheimer's Network

INTRODUCTION

"We are not human beings having a spiritual experience. We are spiritual beings having a human experience." - Pierre Teilhard de Chardin, The Phenomenon of Man, 1955

The older I get, the more apparent this truth becomes: fruitful living requires learning to navigate transitions, so that growth remains a greater force than decay. This lesson is taught via self-knowledge gained through grace in hardship, along with a lot of letting go, leaning on those we love, and loving more deeply ourselves. I believe learning this truth also requires that we develop (or maintain) spiritual awareness. Otherwise, when confronted with death, life becomes meaningless for us.

Few things in our shared experience are more certain than the changing of seasons. We seem to know in the very chemical bonds of our DNA that spring will follow winter, no matter how cold and gray everything appears. In all seasons, life lies pulsing underneath, poised to shoot out through the cracks. This is reality, and it can be counted on.

But sometimes our perception becomes clouded as we grope for signs of truth on very dark days. Most of us who are caregivers for those with dementia have been in this situation many times. Like our loved ones, we may forget even those things which are deeply known. We can be assured that life always goes on living, whether or not we remember. And to all who can keep themselves open to this truth, fresh signs of that life may be appreciated in any season. Hope renews itself through the sharing of stories—we are warmed to life again by the sun shining upon another.

A setting sun poured out its flaming hues upon summer's distant horizon...

That day was one of the most important of my life. I received a call from my father's employer stating she needed to speak with me. We met in my office; her face was grave, though understanding. "Are you aware of your father's behavior, of his confusion on the job?" "I am not sure what you mean," I said, in frank denial. Dad had recently "retired," but as any descendant of a utilitarian soul can appreciate, remnants of the Great Depression mindset still revealed themselves in his work ethic, which had been honed early on in that crucible of toil known as a saw mill.

He picked up a job parking cars at a medical office building. Sure, there had been signs...a fender bender or two, missed bill payments, short-term memory loss, all of which I chalked up to a recent surgery and move. But I found out he had been locking keys in cars, forgetting where he had parked them, and wandering around, lost in the parking deck. This man, always a favorite co-worker, now found himself among the disgruntled who were having to take up his slack.

"We are going to have to let him go...I am so sorry. I truly understand," she admitted. "My father had dementia, and I think yours does, too." The irony hit me hard. This neurologist had to be told his own father likely had dementia. How could I have failed like this, both personally and professionally? Later that day he called to tell me he would not be working there any longer, but instead, had decided to enjoy his retirement with Mother. "I think that is a wise decision, Dad. You have worked awfully hard all of your life, and so has Mother. You both deserve a rest. Enjoy it!" I hung up and cried. And he hung up and cried.

The first chill of winter's wind whistled beneath the eaves…

The descent was terrifyingly fast. Dad knew he was fading. He stopped smiling. A once peaceful man, Dad's demeanor portrayed a persistent underlying angst, and no one felt comfortable interacting with him anymore. I felt so badly for Mother, and ill-prepared, even as a medical professional, to offer her guidance in the daily challenges she faced. Shame, that soul killer, began to stalk me. And I think Dad felt ashamed, too. He had always been proud of his capabilities, his strength, his dependability and his relational skills. And these, like his memories, seemed to be burning in an uncontrolled house fire.

Fortunately, an opening came available at Caring Days (The Mal and Charlotte Moore Center), a local adult dementia daycare center which had been started by our church, and Mother began taking him there a couple of days per week. We were skeptical that he would agree to stay, though we knew it to be a great example of compassionate, enriching, person-centered care which makes the most of remaining abilities and minimizes disabilities. In addition, they had just started art and music therapy programs. But Dad couldn't paint or sing…

The first few strokes of spring's tender, green prelude appeared upon that season's slate gray sky…

A kindly, salty artist volunteered at the center, and befriended Dad. Having never painted a picture or shown any previous artistic interest or ability, the old saw miller started bringing home richly-colored, well-developed watercolors which were expressive of his life story; a story which he no longer could tell in conventional ways, but which he needed to be able to share, just like all of us do.

Over the next four years, Dad painted over a hundred watercolors to the amazement of family and friends. And in the process, he was transformed. In his brokenness, he was met in the moment by caring workers at the center. They loved him as he was, having made the decision to see beneath the façade of affliction to the human core, rich in content and color, and yearning for validation and relationship. They knew the person was still present, possessing a dignity and an identity that can never be stolen by any disease process. And they gave him the opportunity and support he needed to remain fruitfully alive. His affect brightened once more, his communicative abilities improved, and he was proud of himself again. In addition, he became easier to handle, and Mother was given much-needed respite.

The warmth of a late summer sun was felt within the circle of those who cared…

In the process of physical decay and diminishment, Dad was still able to grow. The growth was in the spiritual realm—I believe his watercolor art represents the imagery of a soaring soul, set free through the attitudes and actions of his caregivers who still believed they would find him through seeking a relationship, and were willing to meet him in his reality. They had no preconceived expectations, no measures to which he was expected to live up. Not having known him prior to disease onset, they didn't have to release the mind's image of the person Dad was to embrace the changing reality of who he was at present.

Longing for the green of spring, we may fail to be moved by autumn's deeper hues…

Accepting reality. Letting go. Leaning on others. Learning to cultivate spiritual awareness. I believe these are essential if we are to successfully run this marathon called caregiving. In the years since Dad's death in 2007, life has provided plenty of opportunities to practice these principles, and to look back with some clarity at those seasons spent caring for him. If I could live those years again, I would live them differently; more deeply and more compassionately toward myself and other caregivers whom I would seek out, and with whom I'd share stories and a listening ear.

At Dad's memorial service, George, his art teacher, approached me with the kind of sparkle-in-the-eye look one gives when they know something you don't. After I thanked him deeply for sharing his gift with Dad, he winked satisfyingly and said, "Son, you haven't seen anything yet. Great things are in store. You just wait." Within a month, George was dead. What had he mysteriously predicted?

In an earlier season, George had known hardship, failure, loss and, I suspect, shame. He had died in the winter of his darkness. Literally died. And after regaining consciousness, George remembered the Voice which calls forth spring from winter, speaking directly to him. "I have given you the gift of life. Now go and share your art with others like you." As soon as he was able, George volunteered at the center, and met an old saw miller who couldn't paint. Soon, wild flowers were sprouting from a vessel run-aground in dementia's storm. And for a time, all the world looked green again.

George knew the truth, and therein, the hope that a gift, once given, only grows. And growth in the spirit of love is always a force greater than decay.

Alzheimer's and other dementias are no respecters of persons. They cut a path across all societies, races, religions, cultures, and economic strata. These conditions are levelers, equalizers; and we all become one in the suffering that results from affliction. In this dark, cold reality, how do we share the warm hope of spring which we know at our core still incubates beneath the mantle of a world locked in the grip of frozen death?

We reach out and hold the hand of one whose life is in transition. Then we hold another. We share our stories of having been there before, of having found faith's fire in our own cold reality. And we give the gift of warmth, which grows because it must. It has thus been shared.

The editorial board of *Seasons of Caring* is deeply grateful to all of our writers from varied spiritual traditions who have shared their gifts of faith and stories in this volume. We pray that you who read these meditations, spoken through many different voices, will be given the courage to find growth in the seasonal transitions along this journey of caregiving.

Daniel C. Potts, MD, FAAN
Editor-in-chief, *Seasons of Caring*

SEASONS

SPRING

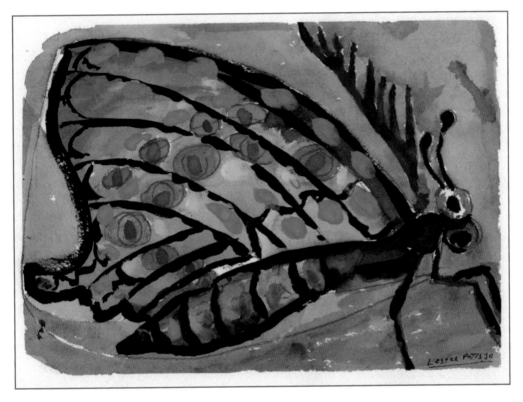

Lester Potts painted this watercolor while transitioning into the middle stage of Alzheimer's disease. The butterfly is a spiritual symbol across many cultures, often representing the soul or transformation. Its life cycle mirrors spiritual growth, and metaphorically illustrates the persistence of life during dormancy or periods of apparent death, only to emerge in a different form. Bursting forth from the cocoon, this beautiful creature finds its new place on the winds in an exuberant dance. The painting was comforting to our family, and gave us hope that Dad's spirit might be breaking free through artful expression and loving care, beckoning us also to join the dance of spring.

THROUGH MY EYES

Do you not yet see or understand? Do you have a hardened heart? Having eyes, do you not see? And having ears, do you not hear? - Mark 8:17b-18a (NIV)

"It is only with the heart that one can see rightly." - Antoine de Saint Exupéry, The Little Prince, 1943

Too often individuals, communities, and whole societies make judgments about persons with Alzheimer's through "eyes that see but do not see," and conclude that they are lost, gone, useless. In order to "rightly" see persons with cognitive diminishment, we need to look with the eyes of our hearts.

Through the great honor of being my mother's companion on the journey, I developed a clear and blessed vision of persons with Alzheimer's. And now I see that they still have the potential to inspire us, teach us, love us, heal us, amuse us, befriend us, calm us, touch us, energize us, enlighten us, empower us, forgive us, nurture us, open our hearts, bring out the best in us, and bring meaning into our lives. With an unending desire—and capacity—to give and receive love, persons with Alzheimer's can reveal to us the healing potential of relationships.

Peggy was my mom's neighbor in the nursing home. Her husband was away for the winter, and although they had spoken on the phone, she hadn't seen him for six months. The first day he returned, he took her out for lunch. When they arrived back at the nursing home, he kissed her goodbye and left her at the nurses' station. With this dreamy, teenager-in-love gleam in her eye, she shouted out to everyone, "I'm going to marry that man!" She didn't remember that he was already her husband, but something in her knew they belonged together.

Perhaps her Spirit recognized his Spirit. That's what I felt happening between Mom and me. One day, I came into her room and she stopped what she was doing. She looked at me—really looked at me. Then she said, "You. You. It's you." It was a moment of pure recognition and belonging, even if she wasn't exactly clear about the relationship between us.

If we can look beyond the losses of memory, cognition, and motor skills, we will make a surprising discovery. Persons with Alzheimer's can still show us the true value of life: theirs and ours. This timeless, human-defining truth is so beautifully expressed in the words of St. Teresa of Avila: "The important thing is not to think much, but to love much."

Holy Spirit, sustain us, please, as we care for our loved ones with Alzheimer's and dementia. Help us to soften our hearts, and to see them through the holy eyes of one who seeks God in every corner of life. Amen.

Rev. Dr. Jade Angelica, Community Minister (Unitarian Universalist)

THE BUTTERFLY

Jesus said to her, "I am the resurrection and the life." - John 11:25

Emily was my "soul sister." We knew each other for 35 years. She loved butterflies! She wore butterfly jewelry, made clothes from butterfly fabric, added butterflies to her paintings, and planted butterfly bushes around her home. The butterfly held great significance for her as the symbol of the Life, Death and Resurrection of Jesus Christ.

Family and friends began to notice increasing changes in Emily—losing her way to familiar places, losing interest in her creative pursuits, watching hour upon hour of television, and wearing a sad countenance instead of her usual great smile. One of the saddest days of my life was the day Emily's husband, son, and I accompanied her to a memory clinic at a nearby university hospital. When the doctor showed her pictures and asked her to identify them, Emily was unable to recognize, of all things, the butterfly. The three of us sitting behind her in the exam room gripped hands. At the end of the tests, the doctor's diagnosis was Alzheimer's disease. The next few years, the disease spun a cocoon around my "soul sister," gradually encasing her in darkness. At my last visit with her, I leaned over her bed and pinned a large fabric blue butterfly on her gown. As I told her what it was, she put her arms around me and held on for a few seconds. She died a few days later with her son and daughter-in-law by her side.

Emily IS a butterfly—a reminder of the eternal life promised us through the Life, Death and Resurrection of our Lord. We enter our earthly life as a variety of funny-looking little caterpillar-people. Then, no matter what the circumstances—life-changing diseases, poor life choices, unexpected disasters, the normal aging process—we all come to the time when we are wrapped in what seems to be an inescapable darkness just like a caterpillar in a cocoon. Our hope and joy is in knowing that we will break free of what appears to be a tomb and soar toward the shimmering light of the indescribable "I AM" in a new and beautiful form!

Whenever I see a butterfly now, I say a prayer of gratitude for the trust dear Emily had in the promise of new life. I praise God for the beauty and love she brought to so many. Just like a butterfly!

Creator God, wondrous signs of Your love and mercy surround us even in the hardest times of our lives. As we care for one another, give us open hearts and minds to witness Your presence with us. Let our hope and joy be found in You. Amen.

Rev. Donna B. Coffman, MDiv (Presbyterian Church, USA)

IT'S OKAY TO BE FRIGHTENED, BUT YOU'RE NOT IN THIS ALONE

Read Genesis, Chapter 3

In Genesis, Adam and Eve eat from the tree of knowledge, and God tells Eve that in consequence, "In pain shall you bear children." To Adam God says, "By the sweat of your brow shall you get bread to eat."

The Jewish tradition teaches that humankind must partner with God in the continuing act of creation. It is our job to recreate this world—with God's help and guidance—to make this world as pleasant, peaceful, and pain-free as it was in the Garden of Eden. Jews call this partnering with God "Tikkun Olam," which means "Repair of the World."

We look to both God and science for hope for the future. Humankind has begun to take on the challenge of Tikkun Olam: epidurals allow women to give birth without pain. And all sorts of farm equipment allow most of us to eat our bread without sweating in the fields to grow our grains. We are making progress toward Eden.

In this day and age, we face challenges the Bible doesn't mention, including brain diseases such as Alzheimer's. Many individuals are diagnosed with Alzheimer's and other dementias, but many more suffer with and because of it: not just the person with the disease, but also that person's family, friends, and caregivers.

My memories of Joe always tear at my heart, and his story typifies Alzheimer's disease. Joe was a gentle, loving man. He was concerned about his appearance and always impeccably dressed. He worked hard all his life, saved his money, and he and his wife dreamed of the day when he would finally be able to retire and they would travel around the world. Their children were grown and raising children of their own when Joe was diagnosed with Alzheimer's. Joe—this sweet and elegant man—became untidy, refused to wash, and would fight his caregivers whenever they tried to get him up from his bed. Joe's wife's dreams of travel with her life partner by her side would remain dreams forever.

In our perception, our hopes and dreams and those of our loved ones seem to disappear slowly until they vanish altogether, until we must grieve over someone whom we feel is no longer with us, someone we may believe we have lost even when their bodies may still be alive. This future can truly be frightening. Fortunately, however, we don't have to go it alone, because caregiving and Tikkun Olam are jobs for the global village.

Let us praise God for the ability to remember, for the hope and promise of the future, when Alzheimer's may itself be but a memory. Let us help repair the world by supporting the work to conquer this and other dementias, by educating those who are in power and those who hold the purse strings. Amen.

Rabbi Susan S. Conforti (Jewish)

YOU CAN NEVER TELL

"In caregiving, it's best to expect the unexpected." - A caregiver

I saw Rose weekly for the better part of a year. She was in the advanced stages of Alzheimer's disease and didn't speak. During the holidays, if Rose received a card, then I would read the card to her and let her hold and see the card, but it was clear she wasn't making sense either of the words her ears heard or the written words her eyes beheld.

As the months went by, I followed a basic visiting routine: after a few minutes of greeting Rose and the staff, I'd give Rose a very gentle massage using a form of compassionate touch that was first used in people with AIDS in the 1980's. After a while, I'd sit next to her bed and read. Or, if Rose was in the living room, then I'd watch TV with her. I had no expectation of providing spiritual care *per se* to Rose because she just was too far gone into the depths of the disease.

One day as I was leaving, I said to Rose the same thing I always said to her: "Rose, I'm going to be leaving now. I ask God to bless you and those who care for you. See you next week." Out of the blue, Rose reached out and grabbed my arm. Then she said, remarkably clearly, "Don't go." So I stayed.

Dear Healer of All Healers, thank you for allowing us to be surprised by people's abilities, even in the late stages of dementia. May we all be privileged to have "Golden Moments" with our loved ones like those I had with Rose. Amen.

Rabbi Susan S. Conforti (Jewish)

SINGING FROM THE SOUL

I will sing to the Lord as long as I live; I will sing praise to my God while I have being.
- Psalm 104:33

St. Francis of Assisi once said: "Preach the Gospel at all times; when necessary use words." In the context of Alzheimer's, it might be said, "Sing unto the Lord with all your heart and soul; when necessary use words."

I've learned from friendships with those who have Alzheimer's that singing doesn't require the ability to speak; singing can mount on eagle's wings *above* verbalization.

Marie is 91. I haven't heard her speak for nearly a year, and even then it's one word, followed by silence. But "silence" does not describe our visits, because silence can imply a lack of communication. That is not at all the case. If "eyes are the window of the soul," then Marie's eyes throw that window wide open. They communicate warmth, joy, gratitude, acceptance, and love.

The first time we met I asked her if she liked the hymn "Great Is Thy Faithfulness." She didn't answer; but, when I started singing, she grasped my hands, swaying them back and forth to the rhythm of the song. It was not me singing to Marie; it was *us*. We joined together musically to express thanks for God's faithfulness. We were singing in harmony—only one of us using words; for the other, words were not necessary.

Louise is another friend with Alzheimer's. When I come to visit, I hear her before I see her, because Louise continually makes a humming sound. I've never heard her say a word, but when I step into her room she greets me with kind eyes, a warm smile and…humming.

One day I asked Louise if she liked "Amazing Grace." She enthusiastically nodded. I sang the first verse, and Louise continued humming—randomly, and with no apparent relation to what I was singing.

Further into the song I noticed that one of the tones Louise hummed matched the note I was singing. And another, and another…by the last verse, Louise was humming every note along with me—on pitch with matching rhythm. We were singing a duet! The woman who could not speak was singing to the Lord with all her heart and soul.

Yes, much is lost to Alzheimer's disease, and the loss continues and deepens with time. But much remains, and what remains is sacred and beautiful.

God, when I look upon my brothers and sisters on this earth, may I see the face of Christ; when I listen to them, may I hear His voice. Amen.

Chaplain Drew DeCrease (Roman Catholic Deacon)

"SOMETHING WONDERFUL IS HAPPENING TO ME..."

Immediately his [Zechariah's] mouth was opened and his tongue loosed, and he began to speak, praising God. - Luke 1:64 (NIV)

There is something unmistakably sacred about communicating with a person who has Alzheimer's disease. Perhaps it is because the ability to speak has been lessened, or is gone altogether, that makes what remains so precious. As a hospice chaplain, I've been amazed time and again when someone who rarely speaks suddenly has a lot to say!

Clarisse is a dear woman with Alzheimer's who I always look forward to seeing. She and I share a love of old-time hymns and country music. Clarisse typically speaks just a few words; she begins with the word "Yes," but struggles to generate more words to express her thoughts.

At our last visit, Clarisse was looking at family photographs on her windowsill. She was pointing to them, trying to talk about her children and grandchildren, but the words just would not come out.

"Would you like to sing with me?" I asked. "Yes." We began with "The Old Rugged Cross." Clarisse just listened and smiled through the first verse, and then at the chorus began to join in: "So I'll cherish the old rugged cross, 'til my trophies at last I lay down..."

For a brief time that afternoon, songs which were beloved to Clarisse throughout her life helped to restore some of her ability to speak. We moved from sacred to country, and soon she was singing about "the night they were playing that beautiful Tennessee Waltz." Her smile lit up the room.

When the singing was over, Clarisse said, as clear as a bell, "Something wonderful is happening to me." We prayed the Lord's Prayer together, and every word of that prayer found its voice.

I thought to myself, "And something wonderful is happening to *me*, too—I have been privileged to be present with Clarisse for this sacred moment, as the disease of Alzheimer's, at least momentarily, was pushed aside by music, the language of the soul.

There is a spark of the divine in every person, at every age, in every condition of life. That spark shines brightly in the lives of persons with Alzheimer's.

Thank you, God, for You set free our souls and spirits, our minds and our tongues, to offer You praise. Amen.

Chaplain Drew DeCrease (Roman Catholic Deacon)

THE TRANSFIGURATION

I was a stranger and you welcomed me. - Matthew 25:35c

On moving day, if we had feared a fight, the dementia had taken care of it for us. Mom had no idea where she was or why she was there. She once said, "Don't you put me in to one of those places. It's warehousing the elderly." In October of last year, she was in "one of those places." Mom put up no fight; the dementia had taken it away. The only fight was the guilt that I had for leaving Mom there.

It was a Thursday afternoon that Mom developed the cough. I stayed late that evening. I watched the aide care for my mother. A perfect stranger caring for my mother. She gently washed my mom with towels. I wanted to tell the aide that my mom once took to water like a fish, and that she still has a drawer full of swim medals from high school and college. The aide took out a comb and swept it through gray hair. I wanted to tell the aide that Mom's hair was as dark as her eyes. When Mom and Dad would go out on dates, she looked like a movie star! I wanted to tell the aide that this one she was tucking into bed used to tuck me into bed on countless occasions, sealing the whole event with a kiss. I wanted to tell this stranger about this stranger who was my mother; but as it was, the aide did not know. She did not need to know.

I stayed with Mom that evening, much later than I thought. I had fallen asleep in the chair and had awakened to a dark room and my mother's heavy breathing. The door opened, and light spilled in across my mother's bed. I recognized her shape and realized that it was time for the late night round. I stayed hidden in the darkness. I watched the stranger pull the covers up to my mother's chin. She raised her hand to her lips and gave it a kiss, and then tenderly delivered it on the forehead of my mother. The aide paused at Mom's bed, and then she made the sign of the cross across her body, blessing my mother, again, with a kiss. The aide transformed into an angel, for surely she knew about the guilt hidden in the corner, a drawer full of medals, dark curls on a Saturday night, the child that is me and the love that is Mom.

Lord, help us to remember that Your love can permeate the darkness with light and turn our dark spaces into Your holy ground. Amen.

Rev. Dr. Donovan Drake (Presbyterian, USA)

SARA'S STORY

The memory of the righteous is a blessing. - Proverbs 10:7a

This is my favorite and most cherished experience with Alzheimer's disease: When I was in college, Sara, the wife of the pastor of the church in that college town, invited students to the manse every Friday night. We would sit around on the floor in front of the open fire, eating popcorn and Sara would read to us from *Winnie the Pooh*. These readings were followed by heated discussions concerning the theology of *Winnie the Pooh*.

Thirty years later, I served for a time as Chaplain at Wesley Woods Retirement Community in Atlanta, assigned to the Alzheimer's Unit. Sara was there and, at first, recognized me and we enjoyed our memories of so long ago. Soon, however, she sadly no longer recognized me.

One night, I decided to invite some of my former college classmates to come to my apartment for an evening of visiting. On a sudden impulse, I decided to get Sara and bring her to the event in my apartment. I placed her in a chair in the corner and the gang sat at her feet on the floor, eating popcorn; and it felt as though we were once again in college. Sara talked and giggled inappropriately. I was embarrassed for her and began to think this was a mistake. However, I went to the bookcase and pulled out *Winnie the Pooh*, handed it to Sara and invited her to read it. She opened the book and began reading with the same excitement and the same rhythms she had used when we were in college. She was the Sara we used to know! When she finished the first story, we were all crying. We clapped, and Sara said, "Let's do it again!" She read for 45 minutes, just as she had 30 years before; and, in that familiar setting, she was her old self!

After 45 minutes, she closed the book, and she was gone again.

I've come to understand that, even with Alzheimer's, many memories are still in place, and in such a familiar setting they can sometimes be retrieved. Those were precious moments for us all, and I hope they were for Sara, as well.

Heavenly Father, even though it is sometimes not readily apparent, we understand there remains a person behind the mask of Alzheimer's—a person who is capable of joy and fellowship. Please help us to create settings to awaken and share precious memories with those we love.

Rev. Dr. S. Miriam Dunson (Presbyterian, USA)

LET THERE BE LIGHT

The light shines in the darkness, and the darkness has not overcome it. - John 1:5 (NIV)

I was a caregiver for my husband from 1997 until his death in 2012.

Dementia is one of the most spiritually and theologically challenging of all illnesses because it calls into question the very nature of personhood, and of relationship. And it is one of the loneliest and most isolating experiences one can imagine.

I've recently reread *No Act of Love Is Ever Wasted* by Drs. Richard Morgan and Jane Thibault. Rereading this book has caused me to ask these questions, "What did I learn from caregiving?" and, "How am I different than I once was?"

When you love someone with dementia, you learn to let go of your own ego. You learn to love unconditionally. You come to understand that love doesn't need to be acknowledged in order to be effective. And once you've crossed this threshold, then you're a different person. It allows for friendships where we don't look at what we can get, but simply care for the well-being of the other person; friendships in which we can express our affection because life is short. To validate another person is perhaps one of the greatest gifts we can give. Loving without any expectation of return can change us, stretch us, and transform us. I think these are the lessons learned and the gifts we are given by loving someone with dementia.

I can't believe there would ever be a day when I thought something good could come from this cruel disease. I remember reading an article by a woman who had breast cancer. She wrote about how the experience made her a more thoughtful and compassionate person. But, in the end, she concluded that she'd just as soon have remained self-absorbed, less caring, less compassionate, and never have experienced the horror of the disease. I guess there are some choices we're not allowed to make.

Transformed or not, I still believe there has been too much suffering by too many for far too long. Drs. Morgan and Thibault remind us that love is not a feeling. It is an act of the will and expressed through action...both in caregiving and in advocacy. We can do better. I hope my advocacy honors the memory of the man I loved and lost to Alzheimer's and shines the light of hope for others facing dementia.

May God direct our advocacy and guide us to a cure and provide peace and support for those with dementia and those caring for loved ones suffering with it. Amen.

Lynda Everman (United Methodist)

THE HOVERING PRESENCE

The Lord will sustain him on his sickbed. - Psalm 41:4 (Tanakh)

There is a passage in the Talmud (Nedarim 40a) based on the above verse that reads: *"haShechinah shruyah al mitato shel hacholeh,* - God's holy presence hovers over the bed of one who is sick."

Now, while you might think that this is telling us that God is always near, even in the presence of illness or impending death, I prefer to interpret it differently. I think it means that when you look upon the face of someone who is ill, frail and impaired by disease, it is imperative to remember; to remember and to never forget that this person is nevertheless, even in his or her illness, even in his or her dementia, even in his or her dehumanized state, even when this person can no longer speak or think, even when this person can no longer recognize you, or can no longer even recognize herself or himself, that this person is still, nevertheless, made in the image of God. Nothing, nothing whatsoever, not even the loss of the mind, can ever destroy the inherent dignity of each and every human being.

This means that no one is ever allowed to refer to someone as "the case in room 503." It means that no one is ever allowed to treat a person roughly or disrespectfully. It means that no one is ever allowed to exploit or mistreat the person who is in their care. It means that no one is allowed to talk in their presence as if they were not there. And, no one is ever allowed to treat them as if they were less than fully human. For, "The Shechinah, God's holy presence, hovers over the bed of the one who is sick." We dare not ever forget that!

May we always remember that each and every human being is created "b'tzelem Elohim – in God's image," and may we always treat them accordingly. Amen.

Rabbi Steven M. Glazer (Jewish)

FINDING OUR WAY

Peace I leave with you; my peace I give to you; not as the world gives do I give to you.
Let not your hearts be troubled, neither let them be afraid. - John 14:27 (ESV)

I remember vividly the first time my husband Hob lapsed into aphasia. His words tumbled out in nonsense syllables, leaving both of us stunned. But twice out of five episodes, in the midst of the aphasia, he looked at me hard and said "I'm clear."

He later confirmed that although he couldn't speak coherently, he understood what was happening.

As caregivers, we are constantly finding our way into new realities as our loved one suffers increasing losses. We need to stay open, free of judgments about how dementia manifests. We become like archaeologists of meaning: we read non-verbal cues; we intuit mood states; we search for meaning in their confused words.

My mother, once a writer and highly articulate, had virtually stopped talking, silenced by Alzheimer's. But one day she looked at me long and hard and declared, "God, physics, and the cosmos."

How thought provoking! Those weren't nonsense words; she had contemplated these subjects before her mind unraveled. Who knows what's going on behind the silence?

We should trust that there is consciousness beyond the brain. Quantum physicists, meditators, and intuitives know this truth. How heartening! For us as caregivers, no matter how advanced our loved one's dementia, a part of them can still hear us.

My mother, silent for over a year, went into a coma the last months of her life. Just before her death, she "communicated" to the three of us who were with her. We were about to leave for supper. With her last bit of energy, she began moving in the bed and making guttural sounds as if to say "don't go now."

We all got it. When we told her we were staying, her face softened. She moved into the dying process and died peacefully about an hour later. Hers was a beautiful death including her amazing communication to us.

Besides people hearing in coma, we also need to trust that there is consciousness beyond the brain/mind, no matter how impaired it may be. Even if no response, even if it stretches our understanding, we can always speak words of love to our dear ones.

May we have the courage to stay open amidst life's challenges and remember the peace that dwells always in the heart. Amen.

Olivia Ames Hoblitzelle (Buddhist)

HELD IN GOD'S MEMORY

Can a mother forget the baby at her breast and have no compassion on the child she has borne? Though she may forget, I will not forget you! - Isaiah 49:15 (NIV)

My dad's wife has Alzheimer's. "Has." Like, it's a condition, a disease, a frightful "has."

I have found great solace from John Swinton's book, *Dementia: Living in the Memories of God*, which rightly reminds us that in Christianity, well-being is not gauged by the presence or absence of illness or distress; well-being is defined by the presence of God, and God is not distant from the one with dementia, or from those who love someone with dementia.

Jonathan Goldingay, an Old Testament scholar, once invited his students to his home for pancakes. He told them his wife suffered severe multiple sclerosis, and she wouldn't recognize or respond to them: "She probably won't remember you afterwards, but in that moment she will appreciate you." Is a visit, a tender word, or an embrace futile because the person won't remember? I have visited people with dementia, and have felt in the moment much love—and have even been ministered to myself because of the other person's ability to love and nurture, even if my name and identity are an enigma.

Here is God's truth for all of us: you will not be forgotten. What did God tell us? "Can a mother forget her baby? But even if she forgets, I will never forget you" (Isaiah 49:15). God remembers us, always. God remembers everything you have forgotten, and clearly. No memory is lost in God; everything that is elusive at this moment will finally be redeemed.

I have seen extremely confused, forgetful people smile warmly and tearfully and even join in singing when some old hymn is played. Perhaps the dementia sufferer cannot pray or read, but the rest of us can for them, and with them.

Lauren Winner tells a wonderful story of an elderly couple coming for Communion. They both took a communion wafer from the priest. The woman dipped hers and ate; then the man dipped his, handed it to her, and she ate it for him. Lauren later learned he was afflicted by a wasting disease making it impossible for him to eat. They were truly in that moment one flesh. Can we be one flesh with persons with dementia?

My dad's wife, after weeks of not saying anything at all, stood up one day and said to him, "All I wanted was to take care of you." And then she slipped back into her aphasia.

A sad, or glorious moment? I'll vote for the glory.

Kind God, thank you for the assurance that we are eternally remembered. Help us to share that promise in supporting those with dementia and their caregivers. Amen.

Rev. Dr. James Howell (United Methodist)

GRACE REVEALED

Amazing grace! How sweet the sound,
That saved a wretch like me!
I once was lost but now am found;
Was blind, but now I see.
- John Newton, "Amazing Grace"

When my great-grandmother was diagnosed with Alzheimer's, I had no idea what that really meant. I was still in my teens, and had never heard of this disease. No one explained to me what to expect about the progression of the disease.

We lived in her house, so my mother became the primary caregiver. Every day we watched her decline. The powerful matriarch was suddenly so small and childlike. She did not always know who I was. I felt as if I had lost my great-grandmother.

Since then, I've learned that it does not need to be this way. We do not have to lose our loved ones to the disease. If we can be open to them as they are in the present moment, then we open ourselves to reconnection and to healing. Our relationship may not be the same, but it can still be rich and meaningful.

Now, when I interact with people with Alzheimer's, I do not see people who are lost, but people who have been found. They are completely in the moment, and constantly remind me that grace abounds in the world.

Holy One of Blessing, help us to receive the gifts of grace that those with Alzheimer's offer us. Help us to let go of our expectations and love them as they are. Amen.

Rev. Darrick Jackson (Unitarian Universalist)

PERCOLATING!

"We sanctify Your name in the world, even as the ministering angels sanctify it on high, as it is written: Holy, holy, holy is the Lord of Hosts; the whole world is full of His glory!" - From the Jewish Shacharit (morning service)

Although it seems to be news these days, I learned years ago the positive effect of music on energizing the spirits of those coping with dementia.

That's why our sing-along group, "The Red Hot Mamas," (TRHM) has been meeting weekly for almost 25 years. Named after a phrase in the song "Washington At Valley Forge," sung by Jim Kweskin's Jug Band, TRHM gets together to sing golden oldies, such as "When the Red, Red Robin Comes Bob, Bob Bobbin' Along," "On the Sunny Side of the Street," and others, with guitar accompaniment by yours truly. Though the playlist never changes, the "Mamas" (and Papas, too) never tire of joining in—by singing and/or tapping their feet. To be sure, it's the latter that I always look for!

One of our "hottest" Mamas is Martha, an African-American lady with dementia and poor vision. But despite her impairments, she is ALWAYS ready to sing. Whether it's gospel music (which she loves), or the repertoire from our weekly group, Martha can be counted on to lend her spirited voice. Harmonizing with Martha on "Bye, Bye Blackbird" is something I look forward to every week. Even in her compromised condition, Martha has kept her delightfully sassy sense of humor. When she starts to giggle—sometimes for no reason—you can feel the energy in the room palpably change.

Once, we were singing a song in which folks were invited to "shake your booty." I said that I would start to shake mine to get everyone started. Martha commented, "You ain't got that much back there to shake!"

However, our best moments with Martha are when she spontaneously breaks into acapella "scat" that channels Cab Calloway and puts anyone listening in a good mood. I feel this is definitely one way that God keeps Martha—and us!—connected to Him.

Indeed, if Martha is "percolating," our TRHM time is sure to be superb! And so, just before we begin, I always greet her and ask, "Martha, are you percolatin' today?" "I certainly am! Praise the Lord!" And I always answer with a whole hearted: "AMEN!"

Heavenly Father, You have created us for Your glory to be Your partners in healing this broken world. When we ourselves experience that brokenness, grant that we still be able to sing, and that our brokenness may sanctify and sweeten our voices. In this way, may we add to the healing, and thus be worthy echoes of the singing heard above. Amen.

Rabbi Cary Kozberg (Jewish)

RADIANT JOY

Good are the luminaries which our God has created... Full of splendor, they radiate brightness; Beautiful is their brilliance throughout the world. They rejoice in rising and exult in their setting, Performing with reverence the will of their Creator. - From the hymn "El Adon" (Jewish Sabbath morning service)

Radiant Joy

With Radiant Joy
At the very moment of affirming
The ONE Who Daily
In compassion and goodness
Illuminates the world,
Renewing creation,
Augusta enters:

She of ravaged synapses,
Impaired cognition, plodding speech;

She of bent frame,
Dressed in radiant yellow,
Guiding her walker
Deliberately,
Resplendently,
East to west,
To her place;

She of near-century old legs
Still called to sway
Rhythmically
To our chants.

With joyous tears
I nod
"Amen."

Master of the Universe, in wisdom and in compassion, You renew the work of creation every day. Every day and in every moment, in different voices and in different ways, Your creatures offer praise to You. When moments that seem bereft of joy and meaning present themselves, may it be Your will that our response will be mindful and focused on the wonders that You show us every day. Thus, may we always be grateful, and declare with your Psalmist: "How great are Your works, O Lord! In wisdom You have made them all!" Amen.

Rabbi Cary Kozberg (Jewish)

BLESSING

The Lord bless you and keep you; the Lord make His face to shine upon you and be gracious to you; the Lord lift up His countenance upon you and give you peace.
- Numbers 6:24-26

I was called by Bob, a longtime friend. His wife was frail and in the later stages of Alzheimer's disease. His message was that his wife wanted prayer, so I made arrangements to visit Betty at the nursing home. (Bob shared that their pastor had not visited in three years. I called the pastor to gently encourage him to visit).

As I entered Betty's room I saw the love and devotion. It was evident that she was well cared for and not forgotten by her family. As I took her hand she gave me a smile. I offered a prayer for her and her family. And then, together with four generations of family present, recited the 23rd Psalm. She mouthed many of the long-repeated and even now-remembered words.

Betty's four-year-old great-grandson was very attentive. I invited him to take the seat I had taken by her side. It was evident he had done so before.

To all of us there was amazement as she smiled and reached out her hand and brought Austin's head to her chest. He obliged. Her lips moved. I could not hear but knew (we all knew) Betty was offering a blessing and her love.

With the family's permission, I took some pictures, which I later shared with them: a gift of presence and love through the generations.

Lord, help us to remember and be open to the opportunities for blessing and love which come from the Lord's most frail ones! Amen.

Rev. James D. Ludwick (Retired Clergy/Chaplain, United Methodist)

THE GREATEST OF THESE IS LOVE

And now faith, hope, and love abide, these three; and the greatest of these is love.
- 1 Corinthians 13:13

A loved one with Alzheimer's may change before our very eyes and become, to some extent, like a different person. We must learn to accept this. We must let go of the person we knew and loved for so many years. The one we cherished. We must learn how to embrace and love the "new person" just as he or she is.

Over the years this cycle may be repeated many times as the person inevitably passes through the various stages of the disease. People with Alzheimer's are often constantly changing. Sometimes they become more loveable; sometimes seemingly less so. But one thing is for sure. We must let go of the previous person and love the new one.

This may be extremely difficult. It may test us to the limit. It could be that the person can no longer remember our name. No longer remember our visits. Our loved one may tell others that we don't visit very often, even if we go daily.

One of the most painful stages is when the person no longer even remembers who we are. Or repeatedly asks about people who have passed away. They may ask why those people don't visit.

This may give rise to a feeling of deep grief, but we have to learn to love again. Otherwise, we will be miserable every moment of every day—always wanting to have the person back as he or she was. Yet knowing that person is never coming back, we must struggle to adapt. We must learn to love unconditionally all over again.

Dear Lord, help us learn how to love and cherish our loved ones, despite Alzheimer's, and then to let go with grace and dignity when they change. And teach us how to unconditionally love the people they have become. Amen.

Marie Marley, PhD (Interdenominational)

GROANING IN OUR EARTHLY TENT

Now we know that if the earthly tent we live in is destroyed, we have a building from God, an eternal house in heaven, not built by human hands. Meanwhile we groan, longing to be clothed instead with our heavenly dwelling, because when we are clothed, we will not be found naked. For while we are in this tent, we groan and are burdened, because we do not wish to be unclothed but to be clothed instead with our heavenly dwelling, so that what is mortal may be swallowed up by life. Now the one who has fashioned us for this very purpose is God, who has given us the Spirit as a deposit, guaranteeing what is to come. Therefore we are always confident and know that as long as we are at home in the body we are away from the Lord. For we live by faith, not by sight. We are confident, I say, and would prefer to be away from the body and at home with the Lord. - 2 Corinthians 5:1-8 (NIV)

When we are young and healthy we enjoy our bodies and are proud of our brains and our cognitive ability to learn, communicate and accomplish. We may feel sharp and ever capable. But if the disease of dementia with its resultant loss of mental and physical ability sets in, we may no longer appreciate these things. We struggle to remember, to understand and even to communicate. Desperate for restoration, we may groan under the weight of dementia.

We, and those who love us, long for something better. It is difficult to ultimately understand and make sense of the suffering caused by conditions like Alzheimer's disease, but the hardships of this life make us long for the peace and joy of the next. Afflictions like Alzheimer's may pull us closer to God and create a stronger longing for a dwelling and existence that will never decay or fade.

Though our brains waste away in Alzheimer's disease and other dementias, our souls do not; we can be confident that something much better and more meaningful is being prepared for us. Groaning in our present sufferings, we long for ultimate restoration in the Kingdom of Heaven.

God, have mercy on your children with dementia. Let the burden of dementia be lighter today while they wait for full restoration, a new body and new brain in a place where there will be no more tears, no more suffering and no more forgetting. Though we hope for what is not yet seen, we cling to Your promises today. Amen.

Benjamin T. Mast, PhD (Reformed Christian/Baptist)

THE POWER OF HOPE

This is because we remember your work that comes from faith, your effort that comes from love, and your perseverance that comes from hope in our Lord Jesus Christ in the presence of our God and Father. - 1 Thessalonians 1:3, Common English Bible (CEB)

How weary is the burden of the caregiver. In Greek mythology, Sisyphus was fated to roll a huge boulder up a hill. Tragically, just as he was about to feel release from his burden, the boulder would fall to the depths below and once again, Sisyphus was required to muster the energy to return to what became his life...carrying a burden he could never have imagined.

Much like Sisyphus, caregivers perhaps awaken each morning to thoughts that the burden of care still remains solely on their shoulders. They muster the effort to bear their task because of love and faith. But as in a marathon, perseverance is challenged, and one wonders if the ability to climb down the mountain only to lift the immense rock of caregiving can last the duration. Despair, like a parasite, saps energy and hope for any future dims like a flickering wick.

In Latin, there are two words that reference the concept of the future...futura and adventus. In Jurgen Moltmann's *Theology of Hope*, futura references tomorrow in terms of what has been experienced in the past. Past events inform future events. Adventus, on the other hand, speaks about the future in terms of what has not yet been experienced. It is the unseen anticipation that a child experiences leading up to Christmas morning. For the Christian, it is the excitement as one contemplates not only the first coming of our Lord but also Christ's second coming. Adventus is the proclamation of a Psalmist who had experienced feeling so low that his countenance was downcast. He heard an "advent" that shouted, "Lift up your heads. The King of Glory is about to come in." Adventus is not dependent on past events to define its coming! Something new, something outside ourselves, something wrapped in bright color is about to be revealed. The King of Glory is about to come and rescue by providing a perspective that is not chained to a diagnosis.

The capacity of adventus thunders louder than doubt. It is the hope that David knew in his solitary wilderness so that he could say, "My cup overflows." Adventus is the flower in the desert.

Adventus is the root word for *adventure* that anticipates a wellspring for the soul and sings, "This *is* the day that the Lord has made. I *will* rejoice and be glad in it." Adventus announces hope that fuels love, faith, and perseverance for the caregiver's work.

King of Glory, come in and create in me hope that is beyond my human reach. Amen.

Robert W. Montgomery, MLT, Associate (Presbyterian Church, USA)

JUST BE PRESENT

And the earth was without form, and void; and darkness was upon the face of the deep. And the Spirit of God moved upon the face of the waters. - Genesis 1:2 (KJV)

My sister, a nurse and teacher, spent many years caring for my mother who suffered from dementia and Parkinson's disease. The last time I visited my mother she barely knew me, but when I placed my youngest daughter, then a baby, on her lap, my mother smiled, the one hint that someone I remembered was still there. I can't imagine how difficult this was for my sister. She once told me this was the hardest nursing care she had ever given, though I never heard her complain.

Later, after my sister had developed a terminal illness and came home from the hospital to die, I was there with most of my family. I remember holding her hand and quietly repeating the words of the Twenty-third Psalm, the only comforting words I could think of at the time. I was not an orthodox Christian, but knowing she was, I thought the words might mean more to her. I only managed a few opening words ("The Lord is my shepherd") when my sister's closest friend standing near touched my arm and whispered: "She told me she didn't want to hear these words at her funeral." I stopped and simply stood beside her, remembering the many times she and I sat in Quaker meetings together in quiet expectation. She said she appreciated not only the time for meditation and prayer but the group process itself when someone would rise in the meeting to say a few words and others would follow the train of thought. I recalled later that all my brothers and sisters had initially gone to a Quaker school, so that our earliest spiritual memories began with a few words of gathered silence before the school day begun.

I think now that just being present, without rehearsed words or rituals, was the best I could offer, and I hope what my sister would have wanted. Sometimes just being present is enough. And that's exactly what my sister had done as the primary caregiver for my mother's last years: just be present. There are times too deep for words, and the most we can offer is our presence—a gift of ourselves. We don't have to perform or read words or say prayers necessarily. That's a lesson I learned at the bedside of a caregiver, my sister. Maybe when we say "rest in peace," that's what it really means, both for the dying and for ourselves. Or, in the words of the Psalmist: "Even though I walk through the valley of the shadow of death, I fear no evil; for thou art with me...."

In times of loss, when I or someone else needs comforting, let me learn to be present fully, knowing this may be enough. Amen.

John C. Morgan, PhD (Unitarian Universalist)

AN ANGEL WITHOUT KNOWING IT

Keep on loving one another as brothers (and sisters). Do not forget to entertain strangers, for by so doing some people have entertained angels without knowing it. -
Hebrews 13:1, 2 (NIV)

From the first day I became a visitor in our memory care facility, I was drawn to Arnetta. She usually greeted me with this sweet, old rhyme, "I love you little, I love you big. I love you like a little pig." When I learned she had a little pig she dearly loved, I felt these were words of endearment. We laughed together and became good friends as I listened to her life story.

I followed her as she retrogressed in her struggle with Alzheimer's disease and I became a constant presence, although she forgot my name. I always gave her a copy of *The Upper Room* magazine, and she would flip through the pages, although unable to read its words. It seemed as if it brought her comfort.

I watched her die in slow motion, as she regressed to an infancy stage. Her only words became, "My Daddy," and I felt I had become her Daddy. There were moments when I just sat with her, holding her hand. When I led worship for people with dementia, I taught them the Indian word Namaste: "The Spirit in me greets the Spirit in you." At one of the last worship services before she died, she looked at me and whispered, "Namaste." I knew, without a shadow of a doubt, that our spirits had met. At her Memorial Service I realized that in my visits, I had entertained an angel without knowing it.

Loving Father, as we care for loved ones with dementia, help us see beyond garbled words and unfamiliar behavior to the real person still there. Amen.

Richard L. Morgan, PhD (Retired Clergy, Presbyterian Church USA)

HOPE FOR MRS. PAPER FACE

For now we see in a mirror, dimly, but then we will see face to face. Now I know only in part; then I will know fully, even as I have been fully known. - 1 Corinthians 13:12

Mary suffered from Alzheimer's disease. She wandered aimlessly in the endless halls of the nursing home, stopping only to ask, "Can anyone tell me who I am or where I live?" Gently I took her to her room, and she slumped in an old chair. I noted a faded wedding picture on the mantel of her room.

Mary's face reminded me of the song, "Masquerade," from the New Year's Party in *Phantom of the Opera*. One song from the opera states, "Paper faces on parade." I visited her husband who lived across the hall. Sadly he told me, "She has Alzheimer's disease and it's so hard for me to talk to her anymore," as his voice trailed off into a cavernous silence. I learned they had been married 64 years.

Suddenly, Mary appeared, worried about her husband. Her one contact with reality was her love for him. She sat in stony silence in his old chair while we talked.

I noticed a picture on his dresser of a lovely, dark-haired woman. He told me that was her picture when she was 21, a gift for him one month before her marriage. I looked into her hidden face and said, "Why, Mary, who is this lovely young woman? Can this be you? I believe it is." She smiled. One of the most radiant smiles I have ever seen illuminated her face. The masquerade had ended. I saw no paper face, but a face brilliant with light. "Look, look," her husband exclaimed. "She smiled. She understands." She knew who she had been and now is.

Months later Mary died from pneumonia. I read Paul's hymn of love at her memorial service. Those words haunted me. "Now we see dimly in a mirror, but then we will see face to face. Now I know only in part; then I shall know fully even as I am fully understood."

Her masquerade was finally over. She was face to face with God, and now was fully known.

Loving Father, like Adam and Eve in the garden, we often hide from You and from others our true selves. Often our identity is stripped from us by Alzheimer's disease. But even then we are still there, and live in the hope that one day we can be who we are. Amen.

Reprinted by permission of the author, from Richard L. Morgan, *With Faces to the Evening Sun: Faith Stories from the Nursing Home* (Wipf and Stock, 2014).

GOD OF ALL COMFORT

Blessed be the God and Father of our Lord Jesus Christ, the Father of mercies and God of all comfort, who comforts us in all our affliction, so that we may be able to comfort those who are in any affliction, with the comfort with which we ourselves are comforted by God. - 1 Corinthians 1:3, 4

Hope. Courage. Strength. When caring for a loved one with Alzheimer's, we desperately need these things.

We grasp at straws in search of something that gives us hope and we dig deep for courage and strength. No matter how hard we try, there are moments when we just can't latch onto anything but pure faith; belief in a greater power that walks beside us at all times. It takes trust and conviction to reach this point; but, until we get there, we flounder like tiny ducklings separated from their mother on a vast waterway.

Over the years as my mom continued to decline at the hand of Alzheimer's, I stumbled many times. Why did this have to happen to my mom? Why me? Why us? Why now? Those are simply questions without answers. There is no logical explanation for this disease and it is something that can certainly test one's faith. But hang on.

Talk to God. Pray for His divine guidance. Find peace in knowing you are never alone and He won't give you more than you can bear. Sit quietly with Him and feel the comfort of His hand.

And after it's all over, to the degree possible, be there to help those who may have just begun their journey. Use your faith to guide others through this most difficult time of profound pain and wild uncertainty. In their darkest moments, encourage them to seek comfort by giving their worries over to God just as you did. When we need Him the most, He will never let us down.

Dear Lord, I have complete faith in Your unconditional love; thank you for remaining by my side during this frightening, uncertain time in my life. Your presence is, and always will be, of great comfort when I'm feeling lost. Please provide me the capacity to reach out and comfort others along the way, helping them to see and feel Your devoted hand upon them. Amen.

Ann Napoletan (Interdenominational)

CRUCIBLE OF LOVE

I remember the days of old, I think about all your deeds, I meditate on the works of your hands. I stretch out my hands to you: my soul thirsts for you like a parched land.
- Psalm 143:5, 6

They were there—seventh row back, same pew—like they have been every Wednesday morning. His white hair was carefully parted and combed, his shirt crisply ironed. She, a petite brunette, sat close to him and held his hand. I occupied my usual place across the aisle.

When time came during the liturgy for the exchange of The Peace, I observed a serene, child-like wonder on the man's face which lit up when I took his hand, shook it and said, "The peace of the Lord be with you." I reached for his wife's hand. Fear and weariness in her eyes led me to say, "I think you need a big hug. You're doing an amazing job taking care of your husband." Tears filled her eyes as we embraced. All in attendance greeted one another exuberantly.

Attending Sunday services is no longer feasible since the husband gets frightened by crowds and the pageantry of a full-scale worship service. But mid-week, with ten to twelve congregants, the couple is comfortable and comforted. They know we love the Lord and we love them—the only two components required for an experience of Christian community. The time approaches when his disease will keep them from coming, an awareness that heightens the preciousness of time together today. The key word here is *together*.

When it came time to receive communion, the woman led her husband to the altar rail and he knelt, stretched out his hands and smiled. So much of his memory has been erased but he knows to eat and drink, and the radiance on his face makes me believe he remembers the Crucible of Love offered in the elements of bread and wine. He doesn't want to leave the altar rail, and she has to coax him to return to their pew. It is as if his soul thirsts for the Lord God like a parched land and now that he has found the well of living water, he wants to gulp down more. O how my spirit cries out to this man in gratitude for his wisdom!

As the service concluded, the sun broke out and began to shine through the stained glass windows and turn them into prisms of colors that danced on the back of the pews. The man pointed and beamed with wonder and awe.

Gracious, Loving God: Father, Son and Holy Spirit, from the fullness of Your bounty we have all received one blessing after another. Thank You for the gift of our brothers and sisters in Christ. Amen.

Nell E. Noonan, DMin (United Methodist)

WHERE ARE YOU?

So he told them this parable: "Which one of you, having a hundred sheep and losing one of them, does not leave the ninety-nine in the wilderness and go after the one that is lost until he finds it? When he has found it, he lays it on his shoulder and rejoices. - Luke 15:3-5

The muffled sound came from the end of the long corridor in the retirement apartment building where my husband and I lived. As it came closer, I realized a woman was calling, "Laura, Laura," over and over and over again. Four of us opened our doors to see who was desperately crying out. A little slip of a woman, with advanced stages of Alzheimer's, barefoot, in a white cotton gown that swam on her tiny stick figure frame, is frantically looking for Laura, whoever Laura is. She is agitated, in a frenzy. Her small, darting, dark brown eyes reveal a deep anguish within her spirit.

As I walked toward Marilyn, I told the other concerned residents that I would take care of her. One of the first lessons I learned about dealing with persons with dementia and Alzheimer's was to "go with the flow," to try to figure out what was going on with them, and then enter their world as much as possible. I approached face to face so she could see who I was. I told her Laura had to go to the store but would return soon. I reached out, took her hand, put my arm around her shoulders and turned her back in the direction of the apartment she shared with her elderly husband, who was on hospice care.

In a calm voice, I continued to assure Marilyn that everything was okay and she needed to go back home and wait for Laura there. I opened the door and escorted her to a sofa covered with pads. A small dog, quite old and blind in one eye, jumped up and climbed into her lap.

The husband looked up from his crossword book, nodded and said, "Thank you. I guess she escaped again."

As I returned to my apartment, I thought about the parable of the lost sheep who now is found, but sadly Marilyn remains lost to a dreadful disease. We caregivers beg and plead with God to bring healing, to find our loved ones and return them to us. We cannot understand what is happening, but we continue to hold on to hope that God will reach out, take our hand and lead us all home. No matter how lost Marilyn may be, God *will* find her. No matter how lost we may be, God *will* find us. Thanks be to God.

Good and Kind Shepherd, support us caregivers and our loved ones with strength and courage. Find us wherever we may be in our daily pilgrimage and gently lead us home. Amen.

Nell E. Noonan, DMin (United Methodist)

LET'S HAVE DESSERT FIRST

"Martha, Martha," the Lord answered, "you are worried and upset about many things, but few things are needed—or indeed only one. Mary has chosen what is better, and it will not be taken away from her." - Luke 10:41-42 (NIV)

The Lord protects those of childlike faith." - Psalm 116:6a (NLT)

I wheel into the nursing home parking lot, mentally checking the time. I jump out while carefully balancing the laundry, three types of dessert (we are long-since past worrying about our weight), *Dewy Melon* nail polish (a new one to try today), and candy and gum for the staff (a small token of appreciation). "Oh my, I know that I have forgotten something," I scold myself as I rush across the pavement.

As a child, dessert was a rare treat in our home. Since my mom's onset of dementia, she has discovered that she loves desserts. Dessert, as defined by my mom, includes honey buns, pound cake, pies of any description, and her personal favorite, a large banana split with hot fudge. Mama's eyes light up as I enter her room and she whispers with childlike faith, "May we have dessert first?"

In that moment, I realize that my mom's request carries a larger meaning. "Celebrating the moment" can mean having dessert first. My mom may not always remember the grilled cheese sandwiches, oatmeal, and repeating list of daily meals at the nursing home. She does, however, connect emotionally with childlike delight in enjoying something special. This story reminds me of the story of Mary and Martha. My "Martha personality" was so consumed with the tasks of caring for Mama that I almost forgot the most important task: to stop and simply "be in the moment" with her. All other tasks fall far behind that one.

Lord, help me to remember that today is more about "being" than "doing." Help me to understand these cherished moments of sharing a honey bun and simply being together today. Amen.

Laura Pannell, PhD, CPG (United Methodist)

WITH FAITH, WE CAN MAKE IT

...And this is the victory that conquers the world, our faith. - 1 John 5:4

I'm a Certified Nursing Assistant working with memory care residents in an assisted living facility. Most evenings, after dinner, we gather in the living room and often read the Bible and sing old hymns. One evening, a new resident, who had only been with us for a few days, slipped in to the room and took a seat. Jerry cannot slip in and be unnoticed as he stands well over six feet tall.

Jerry was a Vietnam veteran and had been a state trooper for over 28 years. He quietly wept and sang the hymns with us. When I decided to wrap things up, Jerry stood up from his seat, towering tall in that living room. That presented an opportunity for me to introduce our newest resident to the others before he left the room. He respectfully removed his cap with "Vietnam Veteran" embroidered on it, and walked slowly, silently in front of the group. "Jerry, would you like to say something to us," I asked...then, dead silence. Another lady chuckled and replied, "Yeah, Handsome, got anything to tell us?" Others smiled along with her.

Jerry dropped his chin, cap lowered in his hands, then he slowly lifted his head, and said, "I have Alzheimer's." Suddenly, all eyes were on Jerry; several residents nodded their heads. Three others replied respectfully, "Yes, me too!" If a pin could be heard falling on a carpeted floor, it would have been heard in that priceless moment. Now having everyone's full attention, Jerry continued, "It is hard with Alzheimer's, but with faith, we can make it."

I was so aware of God's presence at that moment that no other words were necessary. Our residents began to clap and cheer for Jerry as he slowly walked out of the living area toward his room.

This is why I stay with it, for these amazing moments when God shows His deep concern toward these loved ones with memory loss. Physically and cognitively, their brains may be impaired, but their spirits remain intact and are not affected by memory loss.

Heavenly Father, I thank You for Your presence and pray for continued moments like this one where the spirits of all can be refreshed. We all need inspirational moments to press us on through this life, and these dear ones with memory loss are no different. With faith, we can make it! Amen.

Sarah R. Perry, CNA (Interdenominational Minister)

LOVING THE CHILD WITHIN

And he said: "Truly I tell you, unless you change and become like little children, you will never enter the kingdom of heaven." - Matthew 18:3 (NIV)

... for, behold, the kingdom of God is within you. - Luke 17:21 (KJV)

I was recently asked by a caregiver how I was able to move beyond the reality of my father's Alzheimer's disease and cultivate a meaningful relationship despite his losses. I told her, in all honesty, that I had not known early on what I later learned: that personhood is still there, though it may reveal itself in ways which are uncharacteristic or unfamiliar to us. As author and caregiver Cathie Borrie (*The Long Hello*) has said, we should learn to "listen a different way."

Pondering the caregiver's question this morning, I came to recall that the occasions of most meaningful interaction with Dad during his illness were times when I was able to be fully present with him in the moment; or else, when I was observing others attuning themselves to him in relationship. At those times, the characteristics of Alzheimer's disease (loss of memory, difficulty speaking, agitation, disorientation, unawareness) seemed to temporarily fade away. This happened most often during times of laughter, reminiscence, familiar routine, creativity, or play, and at any time of shared emotional experience. I saw it, too, when Dad spent time with his granddaughters.

In short, I think I had my most cherished experiences as a caregiver when I was able to be together in relationship with Dad as one child would be to another, with no expectations or regrets, each true to himself in the honest, playful innocence of the moment. What was really happening, I am convinced, was an unencumbering of spirits.

Perhaps Dad's loss of cognitive function had removed some layers so that his spirit was more readily known, both by him, and by others who stopped to listen. My task was to allow my spirit to be drawn toward his by believing he was present, and caring enough to find him and love him there through my presence as well.

I had to look within, become a child again, and join my father in his heavenly home.

Good Father, help us to accept each moment as a gift in which to explore what it means to be Your children who love and care for each other as You love and care for us. Help us to learn to know and love the child in each of us. Amen.

Daniel C. Potts, MD, FAAN, Elder (Presbyterian Church, USA)

HOPE SPRINGS ETERNAL

For in this hope we were saved. But hope that is seen is no hope at all. Who hopes for what they already have? But if we hope for what we do not yet have, we wait for it patiently. In the same way, the Spirit helps us in our weakness. We do not know what we ought to pray for, but the Spirit himself intercedes for us through wordless groans. And he who searches our hearts knows the mind of the Spirit, because the Spirit intercedes for God's people in accordance with the will of God.
- Romans 8:24-27 (NIV)

Is it wrong to hope for something we do not have? I've asked myself this question repeatedly. I remember as a kid being hopeful a plane would land in my yard so I could fly it. What a silly thing to hope for. But there have been others. I remember being hopeful my classmate, Barbara Worley, would go steady with me until she chose someone else. Perhaps it is only wrong to hope for selfish things. I remember being hopeful I would be elected president before I turned 50 years of age. Is it only wrong to hope for things like this if later we change our minds? But why would we not hope for a cure for Alzheimer's? We may not be able to save our loved ones from it, but shouldn't we at least hope to save others in the meantime?

Paul asks a haunting question. Who hopes for something already possessed? No, we hope for those things which remain elusive, like a cure for Alzheimer's. What Paul struggles with, as do we modern believers, is how to keep hope alive in the face of contradictory evidence. Paul's answer was simple: It is to trust God's Spirit to give us the patience to endure. In other words, if we hope for the right things we can continue to believe God will address our hopes and desires for as long as it takes. *We should never give up our hope.*

Long ago I gave up hope that my relationship with Barbara would look like it had always looked previously. This means my hope was a false hope and not an act of faith. The process of waiting reveals whether something is the right thing to hope for or not. When it is the right thing to hope for, we never give up. Hope then springs eternal, which means it continues every year. It becomes our second nature to continue to hope and believe. This is significant because without hope, we have no purpose, meaning, or life. Hope then becomes an act of faith we stake our lives upon. So is it wrong to hope for a cure for Alzheimer's? My answer is no. I believe God through the Holy Spirit will bring about a cure someday. I hope you will join me in continuing to be hopeful.

O Holy Spirit, we pray for Your help to remain hopeful and faithful at all times. Give us the patience to continue to trust You when our desired outcome or answers remain elusive. Give us the faith to believe in a cure for Alzheimer's no matter what, so our suffering and our faith will produce perseverance; our perseverance, character; and our character, hope. Amen.

Rev. Dr. William B. Randolph (United Methodist)

SING TO THE LORD A NEW SONG

I will sing of your steadfast love, O Lord, forever; with my mouth I will proclaim your faithfulness to all generations. - Psalm 89:1

Music resides deep in our hearts all our lives, and God's praise can be sung no matter what our mental ability. The joy of song remains for persons with dementia. Music can be a powerful connection to God and to others. Music and worship may need to be adapted for those with mental limitations, but persons can tap into its power to heal and express joy.

My friend Ann has helped me understand the importance of sharing music throughout the dementia process. Most Sundays Ann is at church for worship, sitting in the front pew with a big smile on her face. As a former choir director, she has forgotten much about music theory. Yet at the same time she remembers a great deal about singing.

When Ann sings a familiar Lutheran hymn, she is transformed. As a choir member, she needs help to participate: reminders about when to sing and walk up to stand with the choir, and how to open her music. After receiving assistance with getting organized, her singing reflects beauty, joy and grace. During the liturgy her countenance expresses her pleasure in worship, and on her way back from communion she often thanks the pianist for the lovely music. With a bit of help she is fully able to be part of worship and praise within her church.

Ann reminds us of the importance of music in keeping our spirits alive. Long-loved hymns and liturgies and favorite scripture verses that have comforted throughout all of life remain accessible even when a person becomes forgetful. Rituals get through when words don't. There may be needs for adaptive worship. One chaplain I knew shared the value of the "hymn sandwich" in worshiping with nursing home residents. This meant that she would share an opening, a hymn, a Bible verse, a hymn, a prayer, a hymn and so on: music interspersed with Biblical texts and familiar prayers. Because of the familiar hymns, this approach provides moving worship experiences.

Like Ann, we too can sing a new song of God's praise, no matter what our mental status. And in the words of the hymn, "When in Our Music God is Glorified," the joy remains deep in our souls when we glorify God. Adapted worship to meet particular needs can be meaningful and inspiring, and can keep us connected to community.

Dear God, Help us always to sing Your praises throughout our lives. Keep our hearts open to assist those with dementia to lift their voices to keep singing, even in sharing a new song. Amen.

Martha E. "Marty" Richards (Evangelical Lutheran Church in America)

WE KNOW IN PART

So do not be afraid of them. There is nothing concealed that will not be disclosed, or hidden that will not be made known. - Matthew 10:26 (NIV)

Mrs. A.B. came to live at Holly Hall when I was the Administrator of that well-respected retirement community in Houston, Texas. She was the widow of a Presbyterian minister whose son became a physician. Mrs. A.B. was outgoing by nature and one who involved herself in every aspect of facility management. She had a practice of coming into my office and telling me what needed to be done regarding an employee, another resident, or even what should be changed pertaining to our weekly chapel worship. I allowed her to ramble on, taking it simply as part and parcel of my job.

As time passed, I observed carefully as Mrs. A.B.'s memory started to fail and she became more and more disoriented. After she was transferred to full care, what we called the Infirmary in those days, she was conscious of very little that had been a part of her once busy life. I would go in to visit her and she gave no evidence of knowing me. I would begin my visits with the words, spoken clearly and directly to her, "Mrs. A.B., are you in there?" She remained impassive.

One day, I was taken aback when I went to see her and said those same words. Immediately, she replied without wavering, "What on earth do you mean?" Recovering from my shock, we had a totally lucid conversation, covering everything imaginable that was of interest to her. Then, after just a few days, Mrs. A.B. died.

We didn't know much about Alzheimer's in those days. Perhaps we are approaching a time when there will be an answer to such a deeply human problem. We pray for that day to come soon.

Gracious God, hold near to Your heart those who struggle through the confusion and uncertainty of Alzheimer's disease. Bring, at last, some signs of hope to those who care for ones whose minds this disease has invaded. Bless those who tirelessly work to seek ways through which the power of this darkness may be conquered. Through the love that will not turn away from this human need, we offer our prayer. Amen.

Rev. Wesley F. Stevens, Chaplain, Holly Hall Retirement Community (United Methodist)

THE LIGHT OF GOD

I wish I could show you,
When you are lonely or in darkness,
The astonishing Light of your own Being
- Hafiz

Close your eyes and take three deep breaths, in and out…focusing on your heart.

See the light of your own heart. It may be bright as the sun or radiant as a star, as gentle as a daisy or any form it wants to take. Breathe gently into the Light.

Breathe in Light and breathe out Darkness,

Breathe in Strength and breathe out Weariness,

Breathe in Love and breathe out Loneliness,

Breathe in Patience and breathe out Impatience,

Breathe in Acceptance and breathe out Disappointment,

Breathe in Compassion for self and for loved one, and breathe out Judgment,

Rest in the Light in your heart, seeing it gently spread through your whole body,

radiating out and in, out and in, filling you with delight in your own Being

and in the Being of the one you love.

Dear God, You are the Light of all creation. Thank you for the life of the one that I love. I often find it hard to bear the changes in her/his personality, her/his speech, her/his sometimes bizarre behavior. It is so hard to have a conversation. I miss the person she/he was. I feel lonely and sometimes angry with the effect of Alzheimer's on her/him. Thank you for reminding me of the true essence of him/her. Amen.

Terrie B. Ward, MA, MPA (Siddha Yoga)

SUMMER

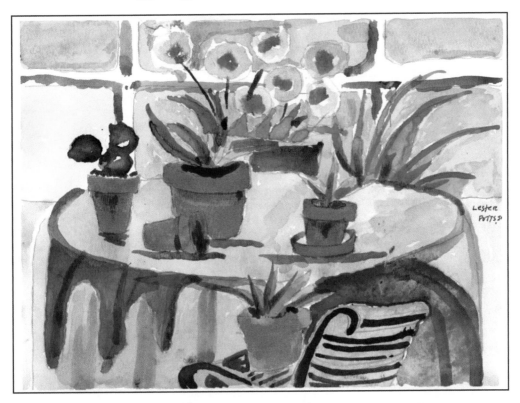

Alabama summers are hot. Lester knew this well, as he worked for many years out of doors in a saw mill. Living things, including humans, tend to wilt in such oppressive conditions, and must be watered often to thrive. This watercolor, painted soon after Dad's diagnosis of Alzheimer's disease, makes me think of watering the lawn and outdoor plants in the summer, and the almost immediate enlivening that occurs as a result. We caregivers must remember to stop and water ourselves on the long, hot summer days, when our tongues are parched and our steps feel like an endless trudging.

CAREGIVER REGRET: A BLESSED TURNING POINT

"To understand everything is to forgive everything." - The Buddha

"For each time that we have struck out in anger without just cause, we forgive our-selves and each other; we begin again in love." - Robert Eller-Isaacs

During the early stage of Alzheimer's, when neither the persons afflicted nor their loved ones understand the changes that are taking place, caregivers may behave in ways that we later re-gret. Because my mother was an alcoholic, her memory had been unreliable and her behavior volatile for my whole life. For more than fifty years, I had navigated choppy waters, and I was on automatic pilot with Mom. As a result, I was oblivious to her emerging vulnerability. This was not the case for my friend, Elizabeth, also a caregiver. She had been joyfully married to her kind, genteel, reliable husband, John, for over 30 years when he began forgetting. She conclud-ed that he wasn't paying attention and she was angry. When he began repeating things and ask-ing the same questions over and over, she became incensed, thinking he was deliberately trying to annoy her. Her response was to ignore him and seethe. Elizabeth and I were both in denial.

Eventually John required more help with tasks than Elizabeth, a very busy professional, want-ed to give. One day, thinking he was being lazy, she snapped at him cruelly, letting him know that he was burdening her. The instant the words left her mouth, she regretted saying them. John's pain shone through his eyes so clearly that Elizabeth wept. She put her arms around him and begged his forgiveness.

This was the turning point for Elizabeth. By allowing herself to see the pain in John's eyes, Elizabeth knew her harsh judgments about him and her unkind behavior toward him were unwarranted. He was doing his best, just as he always had done.

Like all of us, Elizabeth was not a perfect caregiver. She admitted making mistakes along the way. However, because she allowed herself to acknowledge and feel the pain of regret, each caregiving blunder became a powerful teacher for her. Each time she erred, she asked John for forgiveness. Then she began the process of forgiving herself. Wanting to avoid hurting him again or feeling the pain of regret, Elizabeth practiced acceptance and patience; and every morning she made the commitment to—once again—begin, as caregiver for John, in love. Ultimately Elizabeth was able to integrate the constant changes into their life together, and she and John were able to re-kindle their joy-filled marriage. Forever.

Dear God, May Your grace be with us as we face all the changes ahead. When we are impatient or unkind, may we humbly pray for forgiveness. With You by our side, may we commit to begin again, in love. Please give us clarity and strength to do this. Amen.

Rev. Dr. Jade Angelica, Community Minister (Unitarian Universalist)

THE MOST DIFFICULT CLIMB OF ALL

"In the midst of winter, I found there was, within me, an invincible summer... For it says that no matter how hard the world pushes against me, within me, there's something stronger – something better, pushing right back." - Albert Camus

My voice cracked with emotion as I placed the satellite call from the summit of Mt. Everest: "I want to dedicate this summit to my mom and all the Alzheimer's moms out there. We love you, and we miss you..."

With that, the third summit of, "The 7 Summits Climb for Alzheimer's: Memories are Everything" was almost complete. All I had to do was return from the top of the world to the safety of the lower camps in 40-m.p.h. winds at 20 degrees below zero.

Climbing Everest was easy compared to caring for my mom during her last three years with Alzheimer's. She was our family's memory keeper. She knew every detail about the families of all eight of her siblings. She was the glue that held the family together.

And then one day, everything changed. We knew her memory was lapsing, but like most families, we chalked it up to normal aging. And then over breakfast, discussing her husband, my father, who was in critical condition in the ICU, Mom dropped the most unmistakable piece of evidence thus far. "Now, who are you?" she asked me, her 49-year-old son. Alzheimer's had already taken the life of one of her sisters and had a firm grasp on another. But we did not know what we did not know.

Over the next three years, Mom lost the rest of her short-term memory, struggled to take care of herself and began to lose her long-term memory, as well. But she never lost her beautiful personality: her smile, her thoughtfulness, her caring for others and her sense of humor.

She loved music, especially her church songs. She lost the ability to read, so she leafed through magazines enjoying the pictures. We made sure she had her music and magazines. But Alzheimer's takes memories and lives and is particularly cruel. And it may be more difficult for the caregivers than for the individuals themselves.

I pulled the hood of my down suit over my head to keep the harsh winds off my face as I began my descent. My mind drifted to my mom, to my memories. This climb, and all the others, was not about climbing but about people—the need to raise awareness, the urgency to educate, the push to fund research. Every step I take climbing mountains is a step for those with Alzheimer's and their families.

There are plans for us greater than we can imagine. Help us all to use our talents and our resources to overcome the figurative mountains of lack of awareness and insufficient funds so that the next generation need never see another life lost to Alzheimer's disease.

Alan Arnette (Spiritual)

A PRIVILEGE TO SERVE

Read Sacred Songs (Gathas) of Prophet Zarathushtra of ancient Iran

"Brides and you (bridegrooms) pay attention to the words of advice that I, who am encouraging you to marry, give you: achieve a life of good thinking by learning from religious teachings, remain loving righteously (with your heart) towards each other, so that (everyone's) home life will be happy." - Gatha Vahishtoisht (Yasna Chapter 53) verse 5

For many years my wife of 43 years dealt with the challenges of Type 2 diabetes, and she would go to the doctor and take her medicine with my urging. She also worked on weight reduction and dietary changes, eating mostly vegetarian food. But as her diabetes progressed, it affected not just her eyes and the nerves in her limbs, but also her thinking (diabetes is a risk factor for dementia). For instance, she would think that I was doing something with the TV remote or cell phone to irritate her, even though the doctors pointed out that her diabetes was the source of this confusion. As difficult as this was for both of us, I patiently bore through all of that, understanding it was her pain and the progression of the disease that caused her to become irrational.

The progression of her disease caused many difficulties and indignities. Eventually diagnosed with kidney failure and placed on dialysis, she went into a coma due to septic shock; and, after eleven days in the ICU, she passed away.

I tried to keep in mind the teachings to love and be faithful, understanding that the reason for her confusion and anger was her pain and inability to understand its real source. I did my caregiving at home, taking her for doctor's, dialysis, and hospital visits without feeling burdened, being sad but not angry. I retain memories of many happy years we enjoyed together even as I get tears in my eyes remembering her suffering and grieving her loss.

O Almighty God (Ahuramazda) bless with peace the soul of my wife and also the souls of all others who have passed on through difficult times, and give patience and strength to their caregivers as You have given to me. Amen.

Mobed Maneck Bhujwala (Zarathushti)

PATIENT FORGIVENESS

As a prisoner for the Lord, then, I urge you to live a life worthy of the calling you have received. Be completely humble and gentle; be patient, bearing with one another in love. Make every effort to keep the unity of the Spirit through the bond of peace.
- Ephesians 4:1-3 (NIV)

St. Paul suffered a great deal, spent himself fully and gave his all. Now in prison, perhaps he might have wondered why things turned out like this. Might there have been a tinge of disappointment, even bitterness after all he had done? Surely he deserved better.

On the contrary, Paul, who has every reason to be discouraged or tempted to give up, invites us to be just the opposite. He does not feed his negative ego needs. Rather, notice how he goes out of himself, how he encourages us to be gentle and kind to one another, to try once again to be patient, to bear with one another in love, forgive one another and bear with one another's burdens.

At first reading Paul makes all of this sound so simple and yet it is not. When I feel overwhelmed by all of the daily demands of caring for a person with Alzheimer's or a loved one, I need to hear these simple words of Paul. So I read them slowly two or three times, savoring each word until they become a prayer; until these humble words touch my soul and calm my heart. Sometimes I read them aloud. Each time I read these words I hear them differently and often notice something I had not heard in my earlier reading. Paul's words begin to soak in, connect with me inside and calm my soul.

I learn that I can forgive myself for my impatience at the many acts or words often repeated many times. I know the person with the disease cannot help it, but the endless repetition sometimes gets to me. That's the hardest thing of all: forgiving my own impatience. But hearing Paul's calming words helps me to do that: to forgive myself. After experiencing this for a few minutes I am renewed and refreshed. Out of this deep calm I find new courage, new energy to go on, despite how often I fail.

Gracious, loving God, beyond the eons yet intimate with us each moment, be with us now, here. And teach us to be present with You to know how much You love us at this moment. As our Alzheimer's/dementia loved ones teach us so often, we have only this moment, this now. We thank you for the joy and even the pain of this now, this here. We can do no more. It is enough. Thank you. Amen.

Rev. Dick Bresnahan (Roman Catholic)

TAKE COVER

He has shown you, O mortal, what is good. And what does the Lord require of you?
To act justly and to love mercy and to walk humbly with your God. - Micah: 6:8 (NIV)

Mom, Miriam Bresnahan, suffered Alzheimer's/dementia for about ten years beginning in her mid-eighties. Finally we had no choice but to move her into a wonderful nursing facility, a matter about which she had very different ideas. She seemed afraid of the phone in her room and would never answer it, so I had it removed. That was before cell phones, so on holidays, at a pre-arranged time, Mom and I used a lobby pay phone to contact her kids, all of whom lived far away. Usually we would get everyone. Not being able to see to whom she was speaking was difficult, but she never failed to rise to the occasion. One time after talking with everyone, she handed me the phone saying, "Well, that's everyone except that darn Dick." "Mom," I instinctively responded, "I'm Dick." No sooner than I had said it, I regretted my words. I had blown her cover. But she recouped nicely. "Don't you think I know that?" she smiled, laughing and reaching for a hug. She was really good at cover, even when she wasn't good.

Mom had a great sense of dignity and pride. Dad had died suddenly and unexpectedly many years earlier, leaving her penniless and alone to raise three of her six children who were still dependent on her. With a quiet but determined pride she got a job and made sure every one of her kids went to college and beyond. My younger sisters tell of hearing her cry once in a while during the night. But the next morning she was up and at 'em. I'm sure that pride, coupled with her faith, got her through many a tough day. I loved her and respected that pride, that sense of dignity, that perseverance. She never gave up on herself or on any of her family. To do that you sometimes need a little cover.

Gracious God of all blessing, bless those loved ones who have blessed us so richly even when they no longer remember. We do not forget. Amen.

Rev. Dick Bresnahan (Roman Catholic)

MAITRI

[unconditional friendliness toward one's own experience]

"What makes maitri such a different approach is that we are not trying to solve a problem. We are not striving to make pain go away... Practicing loving-kindness toward ourselves seems as good a way as any to start illuminating the darkness of difficult times." - Pema Chodron, When Things Fall Apart, 2000

There may be times, during an exhausting day of caregiving, when we start beating ourselves up, and may find ourselves saying, "I hate myself for doing that." Or, "Darn, I totally lost it!" Or, "I didn't say/do the right thing at all." It may be difficult to accept our own failings and limitations when we become irritable or lose our patience. That's when the practice of maitri is helpful. Ask yourself: "Can I be friendly to this very human part of me? Can I be as understanding and gentle with myself, as I strive to be with the person in my care? Can I apologize if I need to, and then move on?"

When I grant myself the simple grace of being human, I find an amazing by-product: being gentle with myself helps me be gentler to those in my care. And if today I am frustrated with myself or disappointed in the way I have behaved, tomorrow is a new day.

There's something else to acknowledge here, too: the gifts I do bring, the countless ways I am caring and kind and helpful—throughout the long demanding day. But we often tend to take these gifts for granted, to count them only as featherweights—while the few times we "fail" weigh like iron. In fact, acknowledging the gifts we bring to our caregiving is an essential part of having a humble heart. Dear Caregiver, in the midst of so much heartache and stress, hear the voice of appreciation for your faithfulness in staying the course, for your steadfastness to this calling that is yours at this time. Know that you are a blessing, and be gentle with yourself even in this practice.

Please put the book down a moment. Take a deep breath, reflect on this truth: I am indeed a blessing. Count the ways. Now, take another deep breath. Remember that your breath is truly the breath of the Living Spirit moving through you. As is the breath of the person you are caring for. Breathe, breathe, in unison with him or her for a moment. Feel how your breaths become one…

May I have a humble heart, open to the grace of compassion and loving kindness to _____, and to myself. Help me remember that mine is the hand of God bringing the Hand of God to the hand of God. May my caregiving itself be a prayer. Amen.

Rita Bresnahan (catholic)

LOVE NEVER ENDS

It [love] bears all things, believes all things, hopes all things, endures all things. Love never ends. - 1 Corinthians 13:7-8a.

My friend Joan was a gifted organist and served a number of churches over the course of her life. She was smart, articulate, witty and hospitable with her time and her home.

The most memorable acts of friendship she did for me involved her gift for hospitality. During one season in my life, every other month I would make a ten-hour journey to visit and encourage a friend in seminary. Joan always knew my schedule, and on the days when I returned from those trips, I would scarcely have unloaded the car before my telephone would ring, and I would hear Joan's voice saying, "Supper's almost ready; come on over!" Later, she and her husband allowed me to live with them for several months while my house was being built.

There were many other acts of friendship and love across the years, but in later life Joan was diagnosed with Alzheimer's and gradually became less and less the person I remembered. She and her husband moved to a neighboring state to be nearer their adult children and grandchildren, so I didn't get to see them very often.

On one visit, after Joan's condition had progressed to the point where she was living in a memory-care facility, her husband took me to see her. We were both interested to see if she would remember me. In our initial encounter, Joan smiled at me, but gave no indication of recognition. We walked with her around the facility, talking and chatting as normally as we could, and when she grew tired, we sat down in some comfortable chairs with Joan facing me. I noticed that she kept staring at me, and frequently I would smile at her, as her husband and I talked.

During one of the interludes in our talk, Joan, still staring intently at me, quietly spoke. "I love you," she said. Amazed and joyful, I quickly rose from my chair and went to kneel in front of her, taking her hands in mine. "I love you, too, Joan," I said. "I love you, too." Those were the only words Joan spoke during the whole visit, but they were words of joy and hope for her husband and me. They reassured us that in spite of her inability to express herself verbally any more, she was still feeling our love and responding as best she could with her own.

Lord, God, it is the gift of Your love that shows us how to love others. Thank you for the privilege of loving and being loved. Help us to remember that love never ends. Amen.

J. Norfleete Day, PhD (Baptist)

MAKING FIRST THINGS FIRST

Ask and it will be given to you; seek and you will find; knock and the door will be opened to you. For everyone who asks receives; he who seeks finds; and to him who knocks, the door will be opened. - Matt 7:7-8 (NIV)

Alzheimer's disease would appear to be the ultimate loss. The family loses a loved one, a person vibrant and capable, now increasingly unable to interact verbally, increasingly dependent on others to take care of her basic needs.

The deterioration from Alzheimer's is often slow, but it is always unrelenting. A caregiver may be tempted to mark the milestones. The affected individual can get into the car easily, then only with assistance, then only with a transfer board, then not at all; finally she is confined to her bed.

As the caregiver witnesses this tragic decline, she is forced to consider not only the humanity of her loved one and her own humanity, but what it means to be a human being. Perhaps the most noble characteristic of a human being is to be able to reflect on such tragedy and in it find the strength and the means to love, even when love seems unrequited, even without meaning.

I heard a story of a husband caring for his wife who was in the final stages of Alzheimer's. A friend asked him, "Why do you spend such energy caring for a woman who no longer even knows who you are?" The husband replied, "Perhaps, but I know who she is." The husband might have added, "And I know who I am, and who I am compels me to recognize the inherent dignity of my beloved wife, even when she cannot recognize it herself. And my love for her—indeed, my sense of what it means to be fully human—implores me to continue to treat her with the love I promised her when we were married."

Lord, may we so order the priorities of our lives that we place Your will always above our own, and that following Your paths of love we may find You who are Love. Amen.

The Rev. Dr. Michael Gemignani (Episcopal)

A MOST IMPORTANT APPOINTMENT

I am my beloved's, and my beloved is mine. - Song of Songs (Solomon) 6:3

Several years ago, I was at the doctor's office. I was waiting in line to sign my name at the receptionist's desk before I sat down, and I couldn't help overhearing this conversation between the receptionist and the man in front of me. He said to her, "Look, would you do me a big favor. I see that the doctor is running late, and I have to leave in just a few minutes. I have an important appointment, a very important appointment. Could you please get me in early?" The woman said she would do what she could, she would try her best. But then, for some reason, she asked him, "What is the appointment? What is so important that you have to leave so quickly?"

And he said to her, "It's my wife. She is at a facility for people who are suffering from Alzheimer's, and I have to get there in time to have lunch with her."

The receptionist said, "But if she has Alzheimer's, will she really know whether you are there or not?"

And the man said, "Oh, no. She doesn't even know who I am anymore. She hasn't for a long, long time."

And the receptionist said, "If she doesn't even know who you are, then what's the big rush to get there in time to have lunch with her?"

The man replied, "You don't understand. She may not know who I am, but *I* still know who *she* is."

The receptionist walked into the doctor's office and said something to him. Then she came out and escorted this man right into the doctor's office. Then she turned to me, and with tears in her eyes said, "That's the kind of love that I would like to have in my life someday."

That is the true meaning of caregiving.

May God bless each one of us with strength and good health. And if, in the future, we become infirm, then may God bless us with the joy of having such a caregiver as that gentleman, one who is truly devoted, and one who is truly heroic. And, if it turns out to be our lot to be the caregiver, then may we perform this sacred task as carefully, as lovingly, and as patiently as we can. And may God help us in this task. Amen.

Rabbi Steven M. Glazer (Jewish)

THE MOST IMPORTANT LESSON!

"But take utmost care..." - Deuteronomy 4:9 (Tanakh)

If there is one "most important" lesson that I would offer to those of us who are, or will one day be, caregivers, it is this: know and understand that the task of the caregiver is not to cure. Sometimes, curing is simply not an option—not for the doctor and not for the caregiver.

The task of the caregiver is not to cure, but to give to the person who is ill the most valuable gift that we can give them, the gift of reassurance and unconditional love.

Every day we have the power and the ability to send a message to the one for whom we care, whether they have the power and the ability to receive and comprehend it or not. We have the power to say to them, by our words and by our deeds, that: "You matter to me, and in my eyes you are still precious. You may not know who you are anymore, but I know who you are, and I care about you. Despite the damage that illness has done to your body and your mind, you are still precious to me."

And, if you can do that, if you can send that message, as difficult as it is to convey and as difficult as it is to receive, I can think of no act that anyone can perform that is of greater value than this.

Give me the strength and patience, O Lord, to approach those under my care with unconditional love and reassurance, knowing that, even in their broken states, they remain children of God, in whose souls reside Divine sparks. Amen.

Rabbi Steven M. Glazer (Jewish)

THE ALCHEMY OF HELPLESSNESS

"Your loving doesn't know its majesty / until it knows its helplessness."
- Jalaluddin Rumi, The Essential Rumi, Translation by Coleman Barks, 2004

I could hardly believe the ruthlessness of dementia as I watched my husband's beautiful mind unraveling into confusion—each loss another shock, another grief.

Early in his illness, I'd asked Hob to share his inner process when he could. We jokingly called them his "reports from the interior." "What's the name of this disease I have? Horseblinders?" He laughed, knowing the word was wrong, but still conveyed meaning.

"My mind is really going. It's terrifying. If I stop talking now, maybe nothing in the morning either. Depression is right around the corner." By now, both of us were living with increasing helplessness—his and mine.

On New Year's Day, I randomly opened a book of Rumi's poetry and prayed for a message. I sorely needed inspiration. The first place my eyes alighted said:

> *Always check your inner state with the lord of your heart.*
> *Copper doesn't know it's copper, until it's changed to gold.*
> *Your loving doesn't know its majesty, until it knows its helplessness.*

How astonishing! I copied out the verse to keep on my altar. The first line was reminiscent of the Christian practice of the presence of God. The image of transformation—of copper to gold—comes from alchemy. The last line pointed to a great mystery: in accepting our helplessness, we discover the deepest sources of our loving.

The progression of Hob's dementia led to many episodes where we ricocheted between humor and helplessness. He would start to sink into discouragement, and I'd cast about for something—anything—to uplift him. One day he said, "I feel as though everything's over. No more to give." As a lifelong teacher, especially the spiritual teacher of his later years, this was perhaps the hardest.

"It's no longer about the words," I said to him. "It's about *how* you're living now—your acceptance, humor, and lightness of spirit. That's the way you're teaching now. And we must remember the love that's holding us."

His mood shifted, he smiled. The little miracle had happened again. These shifts were grace, copper turning into gold. The majesty of loving—ours and everyone around us—was the greatest gift of his illness.

Beloved One, help us to accept the challenges that are part of this journey and trust that love that will carry us through. Amen.

Olivia Ames Hoblitzelle (Buddhist)

"REJOICE IN THE LORD... EVEN WHEN"

Rejoice in the Lord always; again I will say, rejoice! Let your gentle spirit be known to all men. The Lord is near. Be anxious for nothing, but in everything by prayer and supplication with thanksgiving let your requests be made known to God. And the peace of God, which surpasses all comprehension, will guard your hearts and your minds in Christ Jesus. - Philippians 4:4-7 (NIV)

The concept of leading worship in a Senior Living community's memory care unit was new and unknown to me as a chaplain. Early on I struggled with how to lead the residents to "rejoice in the Lord" when the worshipers suffer with dementia, Alzheimer's disease or other forms of impairment. How does one communicate God's love for each one gathered and affirm the central value of all people and facilitate meaningful worship?

One thing I knew—music was very therapeutic with those in a hospice setting. I learned very quickly that older hymns helped transport the residents to a time they could remember with gladness, even if it was only for a moment—remembering songs and prayers many learned in childhood. Without even having to look at music the residents could recall the words of their cherished hymns.

I am thankful that the merciful presence of God is not dependent on my knowledge and abilities. I have found the music, the biblical story, and prayers we have learned can reach those gathered. Even though they might forget the experience ten minutes later, they still can be moved and touched at some level.

Creating and celebrating worship with this community, I have discovered, can be very uplifting and fulfilling. I have felt blessed by their presence and the worship that we share together.

Dear loving God, whose mercy extends beyond the limits of our human capacity, help us learn not to worry about anything, but in prayer and worship, to give everything over to You. Amen.

Rev. Phil Jamison, Jr., Chaplain, Redstone Highlands (Presbyterian Church, USA)

GLIMPSES OF THE DIVINE

True, True, True is that Lord.
No one is separate from the True Primal Lord.
They alone enter the Lord's Sanctuary, whom the Lord inspires to enter.
Meditating, meditating in remembrance,
they sing and preach the Glorious Praises of the Lord.
Doubt and skepticism do not affect them at all.
They behold the manifest glory of the Lord.
They are the Holy Saints - they reach this destination.
Oh my soul, I am forever a sacrifice to them.
- Shabad (passage) by Guru Arjan Dev, the 5th Sikh Guru

Medical Meditation® for a Calm Heart
(a Kundalini Yoga meditation as taught by Yogi Bhajan, PhD)

Sit in Easy Pose or in a chair with your spine straight. Either close your eyes, or look straight ahead with your eyes half open. Concentrate on the flow of breath. Regulate your breath consciously. Inhale slowly and deeply through both nostrils. Then hold your breath in as long as possible. Then exhale through the nose smoothly, gradually, and completely. When your breath is totally out, hold the breath out for as long as possible. Start at your best capacity and notice how you can slowly hold the breath for longer. Continue in a smooth manner.

Place your left hand on the center of your chest at your heart center level. The palm is flat against your chest. The right hand is in gyan or yoga mudra; that is, the index finger touches the thumb. The other fingers are straight but relaxed. Raise your right hand to your right side as if giving a pledge. Your palm faces forward and your elbow is relaxed near your side.

To end, inhale, hold your breath for a few seconds, then exhale and relax both arms. Take a few minutes before opening your eyes and standing. Continue for three to five minutes.

This meditation brings about a feeling of calmness and clarifies your relationship with yourself and others. If you are upset about something, sit in this meditation for three to five minutes before deciding how to act. Then act with your full heart. This meditation is perfect for beginners and advanced meditators, because it opens and deepens your awareness of breath, and conditions the heart and lungs.

Dear Creator, You brought us here with a purpose. May we accept Your will at this time and at all times, and may we find strength in our real essence as human beings who are a part of Your perfect creation. Amen.

Kirti Kaur Khalsa (Sikh Dharma Int'l Minister)

REFLECTIONS FROM INFINITY

Oh my soul, answer evil with goodness; do not fill your mind with anger.
Your body shall not suffer from any disease, and you shall obtain everything.
- A Shabad (passage) by Bhagat (Devotee) Farid, as written in the Guru Granth Sahib,
the sacred scripture of the Sikhs

Medical Meditation® to Transfer Healing Energy
(a Kundalini Yoga meditation as taught by Yogi Bhajan, PhD)

Sit in Easy Pose or in a chair with your spine straight. Close your eyes and concentrate on the heart center. Let animosity depart, fill the heart with love. Bring your hands in prayer pose, together at the center of your chest. Press your palms against each other with all the strength you have. Try to keep your body relaxed and not tense your neck or shoulders. Breathe long, slow, and deep through the nose for four minutes.

After the first four minutes, stay in the same position and now think of someone you love very much; send them healing thoughts. These thoughts can be transmitted like radio waves; fill the entire room with them, and send them to the person you love. Continue this energy message for one to three minutes.

To end, inhale deeply, fill your chest with love, and project this energy to the one you love as you hold your breath for a few seconds; then exhale. Repeat two more times, feeling energy flowing from your hands to your loved one. Create a mental link. Relax your arms and take a few minutes before opening your eyes and getting up.

Dear Creator, thank you for this opportunity to be the conduit of Your Grace. May we bring peace and healing in our surroundings and always be able to recognize Your Blessings in every situation. Amen.

Kirti Kaur Khalsa (Sikh Dharma Int'l Minister)

"THAT'S MY WIFE!"

For love is stronger than death... Vast floods cannot quench love, nor rivers drown it.
- Song of Solomon 8:6-7 (Tanakh)

Of all the residents I've been privileged to know during my chaplain's career, Tom is one of the most amiable. A quiet man, he always wears a grin. But as easygoing as he is, his life-long preoccupation with orderliness has been magnified by dementia. Now, he insures that even the smallest table crumb is removed, and is often seen on the floor picking up dust bunnies. Tom is also a dog lover who enjoys sitting with his Chihuahua, "Susie," on his lap when his wife, Greta, brings her to visit.

Greta and Tom have been married for 57 years and have three devoted children. Until recently Greta visited a couple of times a week, but her own health issues have lately prevented her from coming as often. It is also harder for her to watch Tom's steady decline. Although a recent anniversary party thrown by the staff seemed to lift her spirits temporarily, her comment that "being here is better than sitting home crying" bespoke a sadness as deep as her love for her husband. A couple of days later, I was privileged to witness a gesture of Tom's eternal devotion to her.

Entering his room, I found Tom sitting on his bed, trying to replace their wedding photo into an old picture frame. He showed me the picture and beamed, "That's my wife!" A missing fastener prevented the photo from staying put, but Tom kept trying to place it where it had probably been for 57 years.

Tom refused my offer to tape it as a temporary fix, needing to correct it himself. He had to do it for his Greta. Continuing at the task, Tom would pause every few moments, look at the photo, and beam again with his original enthusiasm, "That's my wife!"

My eyes overflowing with tears, I thanked him for sharing his most precious possession with me, and rushed back to my office. Marveling at this love that had survived Alzheimer's and would overcome death itself, I shut the door and grabbed a Kleenex.

Eternal Sovereign Spirit, giver of life and breath of inspiration, Your love for us enables us to love others; in so doing, we learn to love You. When life's changes challenge our abilities, may this love remain untouched. Should our powers of understanding be lost, grant that our devotion to loved ones will be strengthened. Feeling devotion's warmth, may our loved ones realize that our affections still abide even if we drown in forgetfulness. Thusly, may we be witness to the truth of Your promise, spoken by Your prophet Hosea: "I will betroth you to Me forever...I will betroth you to Me in faithfulness, and you will know the Lord." Amen.

Rabbi Cary Kozberg (Jewish)

JOY IN THE JOURNEY

"Adam fell that men might be; and men are that they might have joy." - *2 Nephi 2:25*

My husband's grandmother lived in a neighboring city. Through the years I would visit her often and she and I became quite close.

Sadly, we began to notice subtle changes in her personality and soon discovered that she had entered the void of Alzheimer's. Although she had lived alone for decades as a widow, she became as a little child, needing assistance and love as never before.

A caregiver moved in but even her expert assistance could not fill the love that our grandmother required. I prayed for an answer as to how I could serve her so that she felt loved in the way she needed.

The answer that came to me was to bring Grandma a home-cooked dinner several times a week. The homemade rolls, meatloaf, roasted chicken and pot roast seemed to bring her joy, even though she was not able to express it in words.

After some time I had a dream in which our Grandfather (Grandma's deceased husband) joyfully came to me and said, "Thank you." I felt a measure of joy that, to this day, brings tears to my eyes.

Beloved Heavenly Father, we thank Thee for the Atoning Sacrifice of Thy Son, Jesus Christ, which makes it possible for us to feel joy even in the midst of sorrow. We ask Thee, dear Father, to please bless us with inspiration as to how we can bring joy to those who suffer and experience joy as we serve. In the name of Jesus Christ. Amen.

Sister Jill T. Lutz (Mormon)

GET AWAY TO HEAR FROM GOD

Be still and know that I am God. - Psalm 46:10

Where is your quiet place? Do you ever take the time to clear your head?

In the work of caregiving, which is added to the busyness of all our other responsibilities—it's one thing after another. We spend our days caring for another from morning to night; and, when we finally get to the end of the day, we're worn down and turn up the noise to escape the weariness. We can't be still. We can't wait. We can't be quiet. Many times silence is frightening. So we turn on the TV, get the radio going, open up Facebook.

But lingering underneath all the noise and busyness and weariness is a dormant desire to be still and find solace.

I've been reading the story of Moses lately in preparation for an upcoming sermon. God's friendship with Moses began by God speaking to Moses through a burning bush. Exodus 3:1-2 set the stage:

> Now Moses was tending the flock of Jethro his father-in-law, the priest of Midian, and he led the flock to the far side of the wilderness and came to Horeb, the mountain of God. There the angel of the Lord appeared to him in flames of fire from within a bush.

The setting for this great event is my main emphasis. Moses was deep in the wilderness. And, except for the animals, Moses was alone. This was the setting in which God chose to speak. It wasn't noisy. It was lonely.

It was in the wilderness, alone, in the stillness, that God spoke.

The voice of God whispers to us…"Be still. Be still. Be still."

Leave the noise. Find the mountain of God. God will speak.

Father, help us to find the space and opportunity to get away so that we can push the reset button and hear from You. Help us. Turn the chaos into order in our lives. Teach us to be still. Lead us up to the quiet of the mountain where we can hear Your voice. Amen.

Hunter Mobley, Executive Pastor, Christ Church, Nashville (Christian)

FREEDOM: GOODBYE TO GUILT AND SELF-BLAME

"Just do your best—in any circumstance in your life. It doesn't matter if you are sick or tired, if you always do your best there is no way you can judge yourself. And if you don't judge yourself there is no way you are going to suffer from guilt, blame, and self-punishment. By always doing your best, you will break a big spell that you have been under." - Don Miguel Ruiz, The Four Agreements: A Practical Guide to Personal Freedom, 1997

Having a loved one with Alzheimer's or another form of dementia creates fertile ground for intense feelings of guilt, inadequacy, and regret. Caregivers often face a never ending internal turmoil; a voice inside trying to convince them they aren't doing enough or what they are doing isn't good enough.

Throughout my life, I've struggled with guilt about various things, but the journey through Alzheimer's has certainly produced more than its fair share. A thought recently crossed my mind: Is part of my commitment to advocacy and caregiver support a subconscious desire to "make up for" my own perceived failures as a daughter and care partner? It certainly seems plausible.

I cringe when people comment on my being such a good daughter to my mother. The truth is, we had some very, very difficult times early on in her diagnosis. I lacked the patience and understanding I needed. I wasn't always nice, and sometimes I found myself blaming her for not doing enough to keep her brain engaged. I was so lost at the beginning of this journey, so frightened and alone; and, thinking back, I really had no idea just how much harder it would get.

The words of Don Miguel Ruiz are a comforting reminder that I always did my best—the best I was able to do at any given moment in time. Ruiz reminds us, "Under any circumstance, always do your best, no more and no less. But keep in mind that your best is never going to be the same from one moment to the next."

Your best is never going to be the same from one moment to the next. Some days, you will be exhausted or overwhelmed and your best that day will be different from your best on a day where you feel energized and balanced. Over time, you'll learn and grow and that will allow "your best" to shift. In the meantime, be gentle with yourself.

Heavenly Father, please give me the strength and determination to do my best each day. Help me find peace in knowing I did what I could to the best of my ability at any given moment in time. Thank you for your guidance as I learn to be gentle with myself, and please help me to shun destructive, self-deprecating thoughts. Amen.

Ann Napoletan (Interdenominational)

MAKING THE MOST OF THE TIME

Be careful then how you live, not as unwise people but as wise, making the most of the time . . . - Ephesians 5:15,16a

She's a mere shell of who she once was.
I don't visit him anymore; he doesn't know who I am.
Seeing her like this is too hard for me. I can't do it.

Alzheimer's steals a great deal from those it strikes and from their loved ones. It would be easy to focus on what's been lost, but we must remember what is still present and nurture those things.

People with dementia are just that—they are people. Human beings who still feel emotions and need love. Memories fade and moments become increasingly unpredictable; but, at their core, those living with Alzheimer's are still the same people.

Watching a loved one suffer at the hand of this disease is agonizing for us, but imagine what it must be like to be them. Trapped, confused, lonely, and frightened. Something as simple as a smile or a kind word can provide intense joy, even if only for a short time and even if it's ultimately forgotten.

The best gifts we can give our loved ones are those *moments* of joy. Alzheimer's forces us to focus on the present. For someone living with this illness, yesterday is forgotten and tomorrow is beyond reach. All they have is right now, and that might be a lesson we can all take from the experience.

Remember your loved ones' unique character, sense of humor, loves and tastes. What makes them smile? What makes them laugh loudly? What calms them or brings contentment? How do they react to music, gentle touch, chocolate ice cream, or a familiar voice? Pay attention to these things and see what happens.

Time spent together will suddenly feel like a gift. You'll realize beautiful memories can still be made. You'll see loved ones as living, breathing, feeling people who are still very much present. You'll begin to value each smile, word, and touch like never before.

The journey will still be difficult and there will be agonizing moments, but focusing on what is still present instead of putting the emphasis on what is missing will improve things drastically. You'll see a difference in your own attitude and perception as well as your loved one's quality of life.

Heavenly Father, thank you for the gift of these precious moments with my loved one. As time passes, I realize the journey will grow more difficult, but please give me the strength, wisdom, and understanding I need to carry on. I ask that You help me focus on the positive, continuing to love and appreciate the beautiful human being that still exists despite the disease. Amen.

Ann Napoletan (Interdenominational)

THE THING I MISS MOST

Read Psalm 145:8-9, 14, 18-20a

The Lord is good to all, and his compassion is over all that he has made... The Lord watches over all who love him. - Psalm 145:8, 20a

Several of us seniors go to a nearby restaurant after our SilverSneakers exercise session to enjoy a meal and fellowship. During a recent outing, we were talking about the benefits of physical activity and the socialization we share when an attractive, silver-haired woman spoke up. "I would go crazy if I could not come be with you guys three times a week. I need it so much I have hired someone to stay with my husband. His aphasia is worsening and he can no longer be left alone. I can still handle his physical care, but the thing I miss most is conversation. He can no longer comprehend or use words; his frustration grows daily. I get exasperated, too, and my heart breaks while I watch his slow, steady decline."

As we headed to the parking lot, I put my arm around my friend's shoulders. She told me the gift of my devotional books for caregivers helps. Then she asked if she could tell me something else. "This morning at breakfast I told my husband we would be going to a dear friend's funeral tomorrow. I was getting ready to come to the gym and waiting for the sitter when I looked up and saw my husband completely nude standing in the doorway. When I asked what he was doing, he tried to tell me. I finally figured out he wanted to bathe before going to the funeral. He looked so confused and sad that I felt broken to the core. I just took his hand and led him back to the bedroom." She apologized for unloading on me.

It was time for my side of the conversation. I reminded her she was doing great self-care by coming to SilverSneakers and our lunch bunch. I thanked her for talking rather than stoically keeping a lid on what she was living each day. Many caregivers have the silly notion it is a sign of weakness to "talk," but honest sharing is therapeutic. It is essential to open up to trustworthy friends, clergy, and/or professionals who can assure us the Lord watches over us and cares about our struggles. We caregivers are invited to ceaselessly remember God wraps us and our loved ones in love and in hope so deep and so profound it can bear the pain and ravages of any incurable disease including aphasia and Alzheimer's.

Lord God, Everlasting Creator of us all, we lift up our gratitude for Your compassion that gives us comfort and strength for the daily frustrations of caregiving. May we reach out to others to accompany us on the journey. Amen.

Nell E. Noonan, DMin (United Methodist)

REMEMBER

Read Psalm 138

I give you thanks, O Lord, with my whole heart... The Lord will fulfill his purpose for me; your steadfast love, O Lord, endures forever. - Psalm 138:1a, 8a

A caregiver shared this little scene. Her husband has learned to make a grunt followed by a click to get her attention. This morning when she responded she saw him repeatedly rolling his thumb across his fingers so she retrieved a cookie, put it in his hand and returned to the laundry. A brief time passed before the grunt/click resumed. He still held the cookie in his hand but was rolling his fingers on the other hand. He struggled to form the words until she guessed he wanted to take his medicine. He had done that so she gave him a Jelly Belly in his medicine cup and returned to her chores knowing she would be summoned again and again.

As she spoke, memories flooded in of my caregiving years with my husband, now deceased. I became his memory—to tell him he had eaten breakfast, the disease he had was diabetes (he had several but obsessed on that one), the stuff on his plate was called broccoli—you get the picture. I recalled the primary lesson I learned in support group: *Remember it's the disease and not the person.* Remember he cannot help what he does; he's not who he used to be.

One night I climbed into bed exhausted after an especially difficult day. I cried out to the Lord, "I know how Your disciples felt when that squall came up and their boat was being swamped. You simply slept in the stern on Your cushion. And now You don't seem to care my boat's full of water. Wake up, Jesus: please, help me. I'm sinking. Remember us."

I had a strange sensation Jesus entered the room. He spoke, "Yes, I remember, but do you remember I calmed the storm and told my friends to have faith? The Lord will not forget you. Remember God told his children, 'I have you inscribed on the palms of my hands' (Isaiah 49:15-16). Remember you and Bob are sealed by the Holy Spirit in baptism and marked as Christ's own forever. Do you have any idea how much I love you? I died for you. My child, you have been remembered since the beginning of time, remembered now, remembered always. My steadfast love never ceases. My mercies never end. Great is the Lord's faithfulness."

Humbled, grateful, loved...I fell into a deep renewing sleep.

God of steadfast love and mercy, help us caregivers to never forget You are with us in the difficult challenges, the times of exhaustion and exasperation while we provide care to our loved ones. Thank you for the love that sustains and guides us toward safe harbor in You. Amen.

Nell E. Noonan, DMin (United Methodist)

HEART WISDOM

Be aware of that which is right in front of you; then you will be able to grasp what is out of your sight. For there is nothing hidden that will not be known. - Gospel of Thomas

Windows are moments of clarity that a person with dementia has at times.

I have heard stories of people being able to speak to their loved ones at their time of death. I was hoping that when the time came my mother would be able to say something to us. Instead of spoken words, we were gifted with my mother taking long moments to look into our eyes for the week of her transition.

My mother created a bond with each one of her family and caregivers during that final week of her human experience, a bond that will continue to keep us connected to her spirit. She was speaking to us from the wisdom of her heart and making sure that we could see one another and that we would recognize her spirit when we no longer could see her beautiful eyes looking at us, teaching us and loving us. For those of us that were looking, we were able to recognize the individual spark that is her soul as she continues to be present in this dimension and beyond.

When I need help, I close my eyes and look into her beautiful green eyes again. This helps me touch the place in my heart where our souls meet; and, as our souls meet, I can again join her spirit in the flow of energy that is the eternal source of life.

Loving God, help us recognize the spirit of one another. Amen.

Rev. Linn Possell (The United Church of Christ)

THE FREEDOM TO BE

"He who wants to do good knocks at the gate. He who loves finds the gate open."
- Radindranath Tagore

The "freedom to be" is a way that we can bring healing to those around us and is an immeasurable gift that we can give to one another.

We give the "freedom to be" to those around us when we honor one another and believe that ALL life is sacred. In Hinduism, *Namaste* means, "I honor the sacred in you." It does not mean some aspects of you are sacred and other aspects are not. It means that life's essence is sacred.

Healing is a possibility that exists for all life, regardless of circumstance or situation. What this requires is openness, love, and the understanding that the essence of life is love. And, because the essence of life is love, we live this out when we focus our attention and energy on love. Life is not the finite pieces of our individual lives that create the boxes in which we place one another. Life is a creative process that is the ever-unfolding energy of love.

When we make a conscious choice to live in and be a part of this energy, we allow ourselves and those around us the opportunity to live freely, without labels and expectations that restrict our ability to tap into our energy of love. The possibilities of a new life for ourselves and for the people with whom we interact is…a matter of choice.

Creator of all things, grant us the wisdom and awareness to recognize the sacred life around us. May we honor each life and heal one another by allowing one another the grace and freedom to "be" just as You have done for us. Amen.

Rev. Linn Possell (The United Church of Christ)

REMEMBER TO CHECK YOUR BAGGAGE

Finally, brothers and sisters, whatever is true, whatever is noble, whatever is right, whatever is pure, whatever is lovely, whatever is admirable—if anything is excellent or praiseworthy, think about such things. - Philippians 4:8 (NIV)

Picture yourself at a busy airport. You arrive to take a two-week trip with a group of friends. As you stand in line, you notice that although you will all go on the same trip for the same amount of time, the amount of baggage you carry varies widely. There are those who take one carry on for the entire two weeks. There are those who take a moderate amount of baggage. And then, there is THAT GIRL, your fellow traveler who checks two huge bags, each of which exceeds the weight limit. She carries both a purse and a carry on, and convinces the baggage minimalist among you to add one of her bags as a second carry on.

Now picture the baggage as the emotional cargo piled upon us by our life experiences, parents, siblings, friends, extended family, etc. There are some of us who are fortunate enough to be baggage minimalists, but some are like our friend in the airport, who carry more baggage than the average pack mule could handle.

To find peace even in the midst of caregiving, strive to shed your emotional baggage. What are the old hurts you are harboring? What are the wounds you've never forgiven? What are the wrongs that still have the power to harm you?

In the 1986 film, *The Mission*, Robert DeNiro's character, Rodrigo Mendoza, kills his younger brother after finding him in bed with Mendoza's fiancé. Thus begins his downward spiral into anger, depression and guilt. As penance for his crime, Mendoza must haul to a remote mountain community a huge burden, including his dead brother's armor and sword. At the end of the grueling journey, we watch as his burden is cut and falls down the mountain away from Mendoza. However, we understand that the physical burden is not the only thing being cut. Mendoza's guilt, anger, and bitterness also are being shed.

This is your choice as a caregiver. You can carry the weight of guilt, anger, and bitterness on your back throughout your life; or, you can cut it away, forgive yourself and those who have wronged you, and live in joy and peace. This is God's desire for us. If you don't know how to get there, pray for God's help for you to be a baggage minimalist.

Holy God, show me the things that prevent me from living in the fullness of Your grace and peace, and by Your loving kindness, help me to shed those, so that I may find joy no matter what my circumstances. Amen.

Ellen Woodward Potts, Elder (Presbyterian Church, USA)

THE BREATH OF LIFE

"Breathe next to me. And I will capture a piece of your soul along with mine."
- Marikit dR. Camba

It's easy to feel overwhelmed when we are called to care for others. I personally find that I often forget to breathe. Taking a deep breath can relax us, revive us, and help us to find our center again when we feel off-kilter.

As I focus on my breath, I remember that this air is the same air once breathed by the saints, the wise ones, the sorrowful ones, the lonely, the ancestors, the brave and the meek. It is the breath of all sustaining Life. As I breathe it in, I know it nourishes my physical being as the very thought of it nourishes my spiritual life. The breath, the heartbeat, the energy of God vibrates throughout all of Life itself.

It is not just my life, it is all of life—and as it is all of life, I am but a tiny part of it. Yet, I feel this life flowing inside of me and I am filled with the excitement and wonder of what it reveals. The mystery of this moment and the next offer me infinite opportunities to be living in the fullness of Love. I can only do this with my connection to my sisters and brothers in my human family. My breath captures the essence of the human soul as other human souls capture the essence of mine.

As I remember my Oneness with all of life, I breathe another breath, and feel my connectedness with the One.

This is the aliveness that lifts me to joyful thankfulness—I celebrate it and send it out to bless the world. What a gift we are given in this life we share.

I remember to breathe deeply. I am calmed and centered. Nothing can disturb the calm peace of my soul as I take in the breath of life.

Rev. Dr. Peggy Price, Center for Spiritual Living (Interdenominational)

GRATITUDE FOR THE OPPORTUNITY TO SERVE

Do what is beautiful. God loves those who do what is beautiful. - Qur'an 2:195

Help God! - Qur'an 47:7

In a Hadith Qudsi (a Revelation from God to the Prophet Muhammad in a dream) God asks the son of Adam, "Why did you not visit Me when I was ill?" The human being is dumbfounded and in a daze. He stutters, "You are the Lord of the worlds!" God then explains that when one of His servants is unwell, "you will find Me with him." When food and drink are offered to one of God's own, they are offered to God, as well.

This is an important lesson for caregivers of persons with dementia and one that should provide encouragement and comfort. As their loved ones become more deeply forgetful and exhibit challenging behaviors, caregivers may find themselves questioning the value of their actions, and wonder if, in fact, their efforts are making a difference. This revelation assures us of the spiritual dimension of caregiving and the value of every deed.

While Alzheimer's disease and other dementias may rob our loved ones of memory and cognitive ability, their identity in the eyes of God—their essential spirit, their soul—is always present, and they remain persons of value.

It is really very simple: when "one of His servants is unwell" God is with him. And, as we visit with those who are ill and continue to comfort and serve them, we are also serving God.

Sufi Prayer: Favor upon favor have You bestowed upon this handful of dust. Thank you God for the sacred opportunity to serve You. I am grateful.

Iman Jamal Rahman (Muslim)

OPENING THE HEART TO DIVINE HEART

Neither my heaven nor my earth can contain Me, but the soft, humble heart of my servant can contain Me. - Hadith Qudsi (Revelation from God to the Prophet Muhammad in a dream)

Research tells us and observation confirms that it is not uncommon for caregivers of those with dementia to experience adverse mental and physical health consequences such as depression, fatigue, stress and susceptibility to illness. Guided meditation can be a means to provide peace and open a passageway between our hearts and the Divine Heart to help alleviate these conditions.

Sit in a comfortable position and gently close your eyes and focus attention on your nostrils. Become mindful of your breath as you inhale and exhale. If thoughts and images float in, know that this is expected. Allow them in and also allow them out, always with compassion for yourself.

After several minutes, shift attention from your nostrils to your physical heart. Lay your hands over your heart. Your heart has been longing to connect with you! Listen to your heartbeat and reflect on the revelation that God cannot be contained in the space of the earth or heavens but can be contained in the space of the loving heart.

Continue to enfold your heart gently with love as you become more and more aware of this astonishing truth: the Divine Heart resides in the human heart. The heart space is infinite and boundless!

Now, with feeling and persistence tell your heart space: "I love you. I am so grateful. I surrender to you." Please choose words that resonate for you. No matter how awkward this initially feels, continue to plant the words in your heart space repeatedly.

May my words of love and gratitude open a passageway between my human heart and the Divine Heart; may a stream of Divine beauty and peace flow into my being; may my words and actions today be infused with qualities of the Divine Heart.

Imam Jamal Rahman (Muslim)

SIGNS OF GOD IN NATURE

Grass agrees to die and rise up again so that it can receive a little of the animal's enthusiasm. - Rumi (13th century Islamic mystic)

Perhaps the most frequently cited natural phenomena in Islamic spirituality is water, a metaphor for the power, beauty, and majesty of divine compassion for self and others. This is a beautiful and useful metaphor as we think about caregivers of persons with dementia and the challenges they face in caring for their loved ones and balancing their own self-care.

There is nothing as soft and yielding as water, yet for overcoming the hardest elements there is nothing as powerful as water. Thus, the person who is merciful and gentle possesses authentic strength. This mercy can be shown in seemingly simple actions: sitting quietly with your loved one, looking at photographs and reminiscing, reading a favorite passage aloud, singing a song or a hymn, and praying.

The Qur'an offers another insight: water gives life to everything in the created world. Wherever water falls, life flourishes. The person who is compassionate is also life-giving and life-affirming. Just as water is essential to all life forms and causes all to blossom and to thrive, the caregiver who is compassionate can offer reassurance, comfort, companionship and validation to those with dementia, and can help nourish the spirits of those afflicted with this disease. Both the persons with dementia and their caregivers need to find a source of this living water to soothe their parched spirits from the ravages of this disease and what feels like a relentless burden of caregiving. We can call upon God to provide water—spiritual strength—to shift our perception so that we can continue to offer care to those we love.

The 14th century Sufi poet Hafiz uses another metaphor to describe the eternal love of our Creator. The earth would die if the sun stopped kissing her. "Even after all this time, the sun never tells the earth, 'Hey, you owe me!' Look what happens with a love like that," says Hafiz: "It lights up the entire sky." Through the grace of God, the caregiver's gift is to bring light into the dark corners of a life afflicted with this disease.

Dear God, may we experience Your Divine Qualities and the glow of Your Presence as we meditate on nature. May Your Presence enlighten and guide us in our caregiving. Amen.

Imam Jamal Rahman (Muslim)

REMAINING FOREVER IN THE SEASON OF SUMMER

...He took the twelve... aside... and said to them... "See, we are going up to Jerusalem, and the Son of Man will be handed over... and they will condemn him to death; then they will hand him over to the Gentiles to be mocked and flogged and crucified; and on the third day he will be raised." - Matthew 20:17-19

"I am living under a death sentence." These words from a friend revealed to me what I already suspected: his forgetfulness was more than having too much to remember. I wanted to dismiss it, but instinctively came up short with an inadequate response, "We are all living under death sentences because no one gets out alive." Mercifully, he ignored my feeble response: "No, some of us die long before our bodies do." I realized the gravity of his truth. We began to talk about the illness trajectory and what would be lost, a conversation repeated several times that summer. His most haunting statement was, "I would give anything to remain here forever, but I can't."

Summer is a time of growth. Like a summer weed, Alzheimer's grows visible, choking out memory. We can see it though we want to linger as long as we can in summer before its progression sets in. And we do for a time. Once set in motion though, we cannot stop it. We can guess what is going to happen, just not when. So summer becomes holding on to what you can, living in the moment, enduring the losses, accepting the changing *person* even if never fully accepting acquiescing to the changes.

As my mom progressed through her disease, I would virtually see a different person every time I visited. My clergy sister would look for signs of the old mom she had loved. My clergy brother avoided visiting altogether for a time, holding on instead to his earlier memories of her. I grew angry with them both, though my annoyance was just my own coping method. We all wanted to dwell in summer as long as possible.

The disciples didn't want Jesus to go to Jerusalem to be crucified. Just like condemned prisoners who must exhaust all their appeals, or basketball teams behind at game's end playing for overtime, our human minds want to avoid loss as long as possible. It is okay to linger in summer while we can; just know it is only temporary. Summer, like it or not, comes to an end. And just like the movement of the seasons, the loss will come and then the season of healing can begin. We can't live in summer forever.

O Creator God, we know You did not create us to become sick with Alzheimer's. We ask to remain for as long as we can in summer with loved ones who suffer. But we must leave summer behind. Help us to cope with our pain and to hold Your hand, knowing You have walked this road already to Your death, so You may guide us when it is fearful and we don't want to go. Amen.

Rev. Dr. William B. Randolph (United Methodist)

A TIME TO REST

Immediately He made the disciples get into the boat and go ahead of Him to the other side, while He sent the crowds away. After He had sent the crowds away, He went up on the mountain by Himself to pray; and when it was evening, He was there alone.
- Matthew 14:22-23 (NIV)

As an employee in a retirement community, I have watched many couples coping together while a partner becomes increasingly impaired by dementia. As disability creeps in, it is natural for the partner to continue adding responsibilities. This gradual shifting of responsibility to one member of the couple inevitably becomes a huge burden for one to bear alone, especially while dealing with the grief of watching your soul mate mentally slipping away from you.

Part of this challenge includes the need for the caregiver always to be with the person who has dementia. Thus, in the greatest times of challenge, the caregiver is pulled away from resources that might help to rebuild his/her strength: prayer time, family, friends, recreation, worship, and even rest.

Rest is essential, a great God-given blessing. Mental and physical time off is required for us to be our best selves. God calls us to serve others; but, in order to most effectively do so, we must practice self-care so that we are offering our best, with all of the gifts and talents God has planted within us.

Jesus often exemplified this. He gave of himself, faithfully serving, teaching and healing, perhaps to the brink of overextension. While he always responded to the needs presented, Jesus made it a point to retreat for time alone with his Father, resting and recharging. If Jesus, who was sent as sacrifice, needed time away, how much more do we have that same need for renewal so that we may continue offering ourselves in service? Taking time to do things that refresh our minds and bodies is always important, but even more essential during times of great pressure.

It may be a challenge to find resources that will allow you to take time away for yourself, but as a caregiver, doing so is not only an important gift to yourself, but one to your loved one as well. Jesus demonstrated that the time we need to rebuild ourselves is not selfish, but an essential part of answering our call to serve.

Dear Lord, I want to give my best to those that I love. Help me to find ways to care for myself, so that I am able to continue to give what is needed at this time. Send help and rest when I grow weary. I lean on You to lift me up when I feel weak. Amen.

Brenda M. Sobota, MSW (Roman Catholic)

LOVE BEARS ALL THINGS

If I speak in the tongues of men or of angels, but do not have love, I am only a resounding gong or a clanging cymbal. If I have the gift of prophecy and can fathom all mysteries and all knowledge, and if I have a faith that can move mountains, but do not have love, I am nothing. If I give all I possess to the poor and give over my body to hardship that I may boast, but do not have love, I gain nothing.

Love is patient, love is kind. It does not envy, it does not boast, it is not proud. It does not dishonor others, it is not self-seeking, it is not easily angered, it keeps no record of wrongs. Love does not delight in evil but rejoices with the truth. It always protects, always trusts, always hopes, always perseveres.

Love never fails. But where there are prophecies, they will cease; where there are tongues, they will be stilled; where there is knowledge, it will pass away. For we know in part and we prophesy in part, but when completeness comes, what is in part disappears. When I was a child, I talked like a child, I thought like a child, I reasoned like a child. When I became a man, I put the ways of childhood behind me. For now we see only a reflection as in a mirror; then we shall see face to face. Now I know in part; then I shall know fully, even as I am fully known.

And now these three remain: faith, hope and love. But the greatest of these is love.
- 1 Corinthians 13:1-13 (NIV)

St. Paul writes in I Corinthians Chapter 13 about love. In his listing of the things love accomplishes is "love bears all things."

For a long time after my wife was diagnosed with dementia I could not understand why this happened to her. She is the nearest person to perfection I have ever known.

In my agony I would cry out to God, "WHY?" and came near to losing my faith. I don't know the reason this disease struck June; but, in my personal struggle dealing with it I have come to realize that God has given me a depth of love for my wife that probably would never have been possible otherwise.

At one time I would have yelled, "Go to sleep!" when she awakened me at 2:00 a.m. talking and singing incoherently. Now I talk and sing with her, and thank God we can do this together.

Love does enable one to bear all things, even sleepless nights.

Holy Lord, author and embodiment of love, teach us the real essence of love as we care for those suffering with dementia. Help us to keep faith, hope and love, these three, central in our lives as caregivers. Amen.

Bishop Philip E. P. Weeks (The Charismatic Episcopal Church)

TRANSITIONS

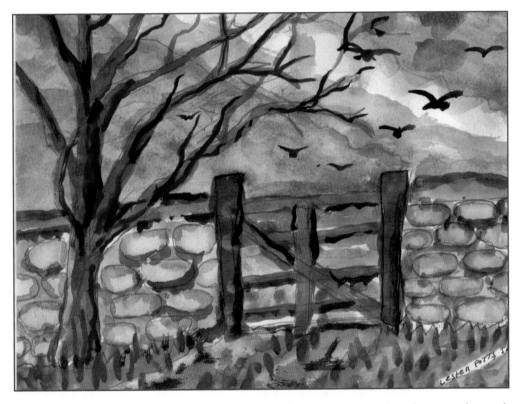

Dad loved fences and gates. He enjoyed building them, painting them, and mending them. He was a man of boundaries and demarcations, maintaining that part for which he was responsible. He never let anything fall into disrepair. Never, that is, until dementia set in. The garden gate had come off of its hinges. Perhaps he didn't notice. I suspect he did, but knew he couldn't make the repairs himself. So I got out the tools and did the job, letting him assist. This was a transition—I had always been the holder of the plank for Dad to do the nailing. Transition can make for an awkward dance as we assume the lead from one who falters, make a home out of new and unfamiliar surroundings, or take away the car keys. When facing transitions we must become fence menders, shoring up the self of the one we love, helping them to maintain awareness of who they are in the midst of change and loss. This, in turn, enables reciprocal relationship... and love flows back and forth through the open gate.

LAST WORDS

"Language is the autobiography of the human mind."- Max Muller, A Dictionary of Scientific Quotations, I. Mackay, 2011

In her last days she speaks fewer and fewer words. It is a reflection of the world she now lives in; closed in, constrained, but also a safe harbor where she can bide her last days in calm waters. Milly is a friend, a good one, much older than I, infinitely wiser, and now we are together, perhaps for the last time in her hospice care room. We had said our first goodbyes years earlier when she had been diagnosed with dementia. Now here we are, together in spirit, even though I suspect that she might be far away from this moment. Where can she be?

I reach across to her and whisper, "It's okay to let go." Milly rolls her head towards me and smiles. She hasn't done that in months. Is she having one of those rare *being present* moments? I look at her again. That beautiful smile, wrinkled with memories and time, is for someone else far beyond me. It is a moment of transition for both of us.

Milly was a teacher and writer. Words were her wisdom. Perhaps they still are, though she has few left to share. It was just one week ago that I heard her say, "Thank you. I'm not alone." Words of grace. Gratitude. Her life story in five words.

There are always sounds, even in a hospice room—the ticking of a clock, the rasped breathing of a body still fighting. Even the quietest energies of life can be draining. Are we in the storm before the calm? Is that what life is, a cataclysmic prelude to something we can only pretend to imagine?

Milly still smiles—now with a gentle peace that comes from deep inside—and she is still here with me. But not for long. I think she has seen another safe harbor, far beyond this one. I whisper again to her, "It's okay to let go."

He stilled the storm to a whisper, the waves of the sea were hushed. - Psalm 107:29

Richard Campbell, MEd (Roman Catholic)

A SONG OF THE SOUL

You are my strength, I sing praise to you; you, God, are my fortress, my God on whom I can rely. - Psalm 59:17 (NIV)

Edwin had dementia, but was still able to walk about his home, putter in the yard, and communicate some of his needs. His wife, Sara, cared for him until the fateful day he suffered a stroke that added insult to injury. It left him unable to walk or talk at all. Edwin could no longer feed himself or help with his bath. He was a very tall, large man so it quickly became apparent to Sara that she could not provide twenty-four-hour care for her beloved husband in their home. She was exhausted.

Edwin moved to the care facility where I worked as an Activity Director. Sara visited him faithfully. The folks who offered his care kept him clean and neat. But they just couldn't understand why they should make the effort and take the time to get him out of bed, into a recliner, and push him down the hall to the Activity Room. After all, Edwin didn't speak or seem to notice anything around him. Why go to all that trouble?

One day shortly before Christmas, I was able to cajole the staff into bringing him to our Christmas Carol party. The residents and volunteers sang several songs. Edwin didn't seem to respond at all. His eyes were closed. Then, when the pianist played the opening chords of "O Come, All Ye Faithful," a new voice joined in the song! It was Edwin! He sang the whole first verse in a clear, strong voice!

> O come, all ye faithful, joyful and triumphant.
> O come ye, O come ye to Bethlehem!
> Come, and behold Him, born the King of angels!
> O come, let us adore Him, O come, let us adore Him,
> O come, let us adore Him, Christ the Lord!

Edwin's eyes remained closed as he sang. My eyes filled with tears of awe as I listened to the song of his soul, "faithful, joyful and triumphant!" He never spoke or sang again. This man with a large body and very much alive spirit died soon after the New Year. Edwin moved one more time—to the heavenly choir!

God of silence and song, as we offer care for our loved ones, help us to remember that while bodies and minds may fail, the soul still sings. Remind us that our own spirits as well as the spirits of others need our tender, gentle care. Teach us to listen for Your song amidst the dailyness of life. Amen.

Rev. Donna B. Coffman, MDiv (Presbyterian Church, USA)

WHY DO YOU COME HERE TO VISIT ME?

I, the LORD, search all hearts and examine secret motives. - Jeremiah 17:10 (NLT)

Search me, O God, and know my heart: try me, and know my thoughts. - Psalm 139:23 (KJV)

Janet was the first person with Alzheimer's I visited when I began as a hospice chaplain. She often struggled for words, but liked to talk about her children, about the flowers outside her window, and to join in a bit on a favorite hymn.

One day I came to see Janet, and she caught me by surprise. She looked up at me from her wheelchair, and asked, "Why do you come here to visit me?"

The question was so direct, and so searching, that it stopped me in my tracks. "What is my real answer," I thought to myself, "and why am I truly here?"

My quick answer to Janet was:

"To be a help and comfort to you…

To join with you on this part of your life's journey…

To support one another…"

And we did indeed support one another; we agreed early on that I would pray for Janet in between our visits, and she would pray for me. I have made this pact with many people on hospice since then, and that gives me the confidence to serve.

But the question is big: "Why do you come here to visit me?"

I suppose I will spend the rest of my years as a chaplain trying to fully answer that question, and to live up to my answer.

God, let me serve and love with sincerity. Amen.

Chaplain Drew DeCrease (Roman Catholic Deacon)

CROSS WORDS

Father, forgive them, for they know not what they do. - Luke 23:34

My grandparents moved from Minnesota to Arkansas, next door to our house. They both did well for a long time. Then Gramma Bea started getting forgetful: wandering down the street into people's homes and finally, setting the kitchen on fire.

There was no other option than to find a place for her. My mother did that with the burden of an only daughter's heart. It was a nice, bright, friendly place and in town near our home for regular visits.

Each day after hurrying five of us off to different schools Mom would go visit her mother. There Gramma Bea would be found sitting on the edge of her bed, dressed in her heavy winter coat with pillbox hat on her head. "I'm ready to go home now, Betty." "Mom, you know you can't go home." "You're keeping me here against my will and I'm going to call the sheriff." And she would. "Yes, Mrs. Daldorff, we'll be there right away to arrest your daughter." The next day: "I'm ready to go home now, Betty…"

At best, as a young teen I was amused and annoyed. Never did it occur to me that my mother was devastated. Like the mythological Prometheus chained to the rock for an eagle to tear out his liver, mom's heart was torn out every morning for trying to help—every morning. She felt guilty for not caring for Mom at home, emotionally drained from the accusations, and angry at her mother.

I wonder if Jesus dealt with anyone who had dementia. Scripture declares that Jesus went through every human test and temptation yet without sin. We know Jesus experienced anger in the temple and frustration with his disciples who just never could "get it." But where do we find him dealing with dementia? Maybe there on the cross as we tormented him…like those loved ones with dementia do to us.

We know they don't mean to hurt us. We understand it is an illness that cannot be reversed. Those around us say they "know" what we are going through. No one judges us these days. But it hurts like a spear thrust in our side piercing our heart, like thorns driven into our heads, like hands pained from helping, like the weight of the world dragging us down. This is the humanity of Jesus. This is why he said, "Father, forgive them for they know not what they do…"

Lord Jesus, in our darkest moments put Your cross words in our hearts and on our lips. Amen.

Rev. Dr. Charles Durham (Presbyterian Church, USA)

CALMING YOUR STORM

Now on one of those days Jesus and His disciples got into a boat, and He said to them, "Let us go over to the other side of the lake." So they launched out. But as they were sailing along He fell asleep; and a fierce gale of wind descended on the lake, and they began to be swamped and to be in danger. They came to Jesus and woke Him up, saying, "Master, Master, we are perishing!" And He got up and rebuked the wind and the surging waves, and they stopped, and it became calm. And He said to them, "Where is your faith?" They were fearful and amazed, saying to one another, "Who then is this, that He commands even the winds and the water, and they obey Him?"
- Luke 8:22-25 (NIV)

The disciples are panicked. Their boat is being blown about by the squall. They're taking on water. Their lives are in danger! And Jesus is asleep. Haven't you ever felt like Jesus is sleeping through your storm? Haven't you ever said something like, "Hey, Jesus, I'm drowning here! Don't you care?"

There are storms we bring on ourselves with our choices and behavior. There are storms that come from being followers of Jesus who are called to push back on evil in its various forms. And then there are the storms that we suffer, not because of anything we have done, not because of anything God has asked us to do, but because we live in a world where the negligence and selfishness of others' decisions fall on us. And we live in a world where we don't yet have cures for every ill.

You might end up going through your storm for a long time until you realize that the only way for calm and order to return is to trust that God is with you. Not gone. Not sleeping, but with you, in the boat with you, and caring about you.

In the middle of the storm, when you trust in Jesus, you don't wear yourself out in panic and complaint. You call on your brothers and sisters to pray with you, to help you listen to what God has for you.

In the middle of the storm, when you trust in Jesus, you call on His name for protection from the enemy, who will whisper words of despair and turn faith into a pitifully small thing to be tossed overboard.

In the middle of the storm, when you trust in Jesus, you can keep the other side of the lake in sight. You trust that the storm will pass over.

In the middle of the storm, when you trust in Jesus—you anticipate having a testimony of how Jesus was with you through the whole thing. Jesus never promised that life would be without storms. But He did promise that He would be with us.

Jesus, be with me in this storm. Calm my panic. Help me hang on. Give me the courage to face today, and the faith to look toward tomorrow. Amen.

Rev. Paige Eaves (United Methodist)

BEYOND THE SURFACE

But Peter said, "I have no silver or gold, but what I have I give you; in the name of Jesus Christ of Nazareth, stand up and walk." - Acts 3:6

This poor man was totally dependent on strangers for every aspect of his life from transportation to providing sustenance. In this state, he could only beg for what he felt he needed in order to survive. Then, one day, he had a chance encounter with two very special people. He made a request of the two men which they could not fill. Here is a summary of that meeting:

The Request: "May I have some money?"

The Reply: "I don't have that. But I am willing to share something else with you."

The Result: A changed life and countenance.

While I'm fairly certain none of us have been given the power to heal the many forms of dementia, we do have some control over difficult situations. How do we handle what seem to be impossible requests from our loved ones? We can do this by focusing on the underlying needs, not the symptoms, and not the literal "asks."

A request from one's parents or a spouse usually signifies a need for comfort. A desire to return to a previous occupation or chore usually signifies a need for meaningful activity. The insistence to return home is, again, a cry for comfort, for what is known and what is familiar. An angry or uncomfortable loved one usually needs soothing or relief. When the need is met and the person reassured, the problem usually goes away. Let us remember to look beyond the surface and see the need.

Father God, as You have done with us, bless us to look beyond the fault and to recognize and do our best to see and meet the needs of those for whom we love and care; in Jesus' name. Amen.

Pastor Bobby Fields, Jr. (Baptist)

FEELING THE LOVE

And now faith, hope, and love abide, these three; and the greatest of these is love.
- I Corinthians 13:13

In his first letter to the Corinthians, the apostle Paul noted that they were spiritually gifted with sound doctrine and numerous gifts of the Spirit; and that they had a working knowledge of what to do. However, without love, all of their actions were futile. They could check things off of a list but they had fallen short of the true meaning of love. Love goes beyond knowledge, mere words, and good deeds. Without a genuine concern for those to whom they ministered, their work was pointless. The same is true for us.

As an Alzheimer's trainer, I have spoken to numerous caregivers who have a working knowledge of dementia and who have memorized advice given during our many workshops and seminars. Some of them have, misguidedly, forced their loved ones to "have fun" with them by trying to doing familiar activities. It was important to the caregiver that the person with dementia still do the things they once enjoyed at the same level at which they once enjoyed them. Perhaps they did this to preserve the illusion that things were still okay. Perhaps they did this because the sorrow of accepting that things had changed was too difficult to internalize. For whatever reasons, this approach almost always leads to an agitated person with dementia and an equally frustrated caregiver.

Remember to take the time to emotionally connect with your loved one. If it means sitting down and watching a favorite show or making a mess in the kitchen, then so be it. Make sure to enjoy the moment more than the activity. The process is what's important.

As a colleague once shared with me, "The person with dementia may not remember who you are, what you said, or what you believe. But they will always remember how you made them feel."

Lord God, as we continue through this day, bestow upon us the gift of acceptance and help us to meet our loved ones where they are today; then bless us to love with the same tender, abiding love and concern that You have for us. It is in Jesus' name that I pray. Amen.

Pastor Bobby Fields, Jr. (Baptist)

WHAT IS TRULY REAL?

God saw all that he had made, and it was very good. - Genesis 1:31 (NIV)

Alzheimer's is a tragic disease, but it is one of the most interesting because the affected person is so often unpredictable. Answers to questions and reactions to events may vary from day to day, or even hour to hour. If the caregiver can keep a sense of humor, not always an easy task, companionship can be amusing, even joy-giving at times. Conversing with a person who has Alzheimer's can also be quite challenging because the caregiver must enter the world of the affected individual. One should not tell people with Alzheimer's that they are wrong. One must share their imagination and respond appropriately within the context of their view of reality. And one may sometimes wonder whose view of reality is the more real.

Indeed, Alzheimer's may (should) make us examine our view of reality, not superficial reality, but reality at its deepest level. Some believe that change is an illusion and the source of suffering. If we can detach ourselves from change, we will achieve peace. But life is filled with changes, and caring for a person with Alzheimer's brings constant change as the caregiver tries to adjust to a kaleidoscope of illusions, physical issues, and negotiating a health care system that itself is constantly in flux.

I believe there is a reality that lies beneath the veneer of change in which we live. I call this reality Love. Once we have embraced Love and embed it in all we do, we will find peace, and it is only in Love that we can find true peace. The world around us changes endlessly, but Love is constant and eternal.

Lord, teach us to love. Help us to see clearly what is most important in Your sight and then to conform our wills to Yours, for it is only in following Your way, the way of love, that we can find true fulfillment and peace even in the most tragic circumstances of our lives. Amen.

The Rev. Dr. Michael Gemignani (Episcopal)

"THE GRACE OF DIMINISHMENT"

"I thank God also for what I call the grace of diminishment." - Pierre Teilhard de Chardin, as quoted in a letter, September 1989

Many years ago, my beloved older friend Mary, then living with cancer, shared a compelling quotation from the French theologian and mystic, Pierre Teilhard de Chardin. "In my younger years, I thanked God for my expanding growing life; but now, in my later years when I find my physical powers growing less, I thank God also for what I call the grace of diminishment."

Many years later as I dealt with the challenges of my husband Hob's dementia, these four words—the grace of diminishment—assumed the power of a mantra. I took refuge in them, remembering that hard as this journey was, at some ultimate level, it was in the natural order of things.

But where is grace in diminishment? Together we opened to new ways of being together. More silence. More touch. More music. More poetry—his great love that remained into his last year.

Hob taught me to slow down. "This stage of life is all about "slowth"—about getting *down* to speed." He laughed; it sounded like "sloth," both languidness and sloths who indeed go *very* slowly. Worlds open up when we slow down. With expanded time, we experience life more fully, more tenderly, and yes, more painfully. Yet pain opens the heart of love. That too is grace.

Fragments of meaning sometimes come through in spite of lost words. As caregivers we need to be receptive to hidden meanings. In the last two months, Hob managed to convey messages that were like premonitions:

"I just wish I could go into the light," he said, a surprisingly complete sentence.

Although he could no longer find many words, his memory for poetry conveyed his meaning:

"I warmed both hands against the fire of life; It sinks and I am ready to depart."

These were moments of grace. And yes, the heartbreak was right there too. Can we be open to both? Can we have faith that even dementia—this most difficult journey—can reveal depths of loving that we couldn't have imagined?

May we cultivate acceptance and trust in the power of grace.

Olivia Ames Hoblitzelle (Buddhist)

DADDY'S GIRL

I sought the LORD, and He answered me, and delivered me from all my fears. They looked to Him and were radiant, and their faces will never be ashamed. This poor man cried, and the LORD heard him and saved him out of all his troubles.
- Psalm 34:4-6 (NIV)

When I was a child, I talked like a child, I thought like a child, I reasoned like a child. When I became a man (woman), I put the ways of childhood behind me.
- 1 Corinthians 13:11 (NIV)

I was between five and six years old when my father had his first episode: a heart attack. A couple of years later that attack was followed by a stroke in his left eye. I learned at an early age that Daddy was not invincible. I would wake up in the middle of the night to crawl into bed with my parents just to make sure his heart was pumping. I loved my daddy. That love caused me to fear, every day, that I might lose him. I struggled because my young mind could not comprehend all that was happening.

I remember when I got sick my dad would just sit with me. He would watch over me like all good parents do. There were times he worried so much he wouldn't let me out of his sight. As much as I feared for him, he feared far more for me when I was not feeling well or when I was hurt.

Later in life my daddy developed emphysema, the result of 50 plus years of smoking. Parkinson's disease was also a demon he fought. Life was becoming a painful road with many challenges. Our family had our hands full for over ten years.

My sister called the day after this past Easter. It appeared he'd had a stroke, was paralyzed on the right and couldn't speak or swallow. Fear swirled in my heart—I headed home and spent as much of the next three-and-a-half weeks with him as possible. I watched over him like he had with me so many times. I fed him, brushed his dentures, laughed with him, and cried for him. But the fears I felt as a child subsided and I knew there was a greater healing to come.

The Divine Parent filled that room every moment. Just as my daddy and I had watched over one another, God kept watch over both of us. As we lived our goodbyes, God held all of us. In those hands we found compassion and courage. On May 8th I sat with Dad as he transitioned to life eternal. *Thanks be to God, my daddy shines in God's presence and he is saved from every trouble.*

Loving, healing God, we know that fear is a part of being human because we do not fully understand how life and death work. But we trust in You to handle our fears as we care for those whom we love. Give us courage to do all that must be done, as well as courage to laugh and cry. We put all our trust in You. Amen.

Rev. Asa H. Majors (United Methodist)

HELP ME SEE THE ROSES

"The optimist sees the rose and not its thorns; the pessimist stares at the thorns, oblivious of the rose." - Kahlil Gibran

John is distraught when he visits his wife, Jean. First of all, he finds the facility depressing. While walking to his wife's room, he passes several residents sitting in wheelchairs. Most are either staring into space or else their heads are hanging down and they appear to be dozing. *What a waste of human life,* he thinks.

Worse still is his wife's condition. She can't bathe or dress herself. She needs help eating. She carries a baby doll around with her everywhere she goes. She acts as though it's a real baby. He has tried and tried to convince her it's just a doll, and he's tried to get her to give it up. All to no avail. John sees only thorns everywhere he looks.

Jill is another regular visitor to the facility. Her mother, the past president of a major university, is in a wheelchair and can often be found playing Bingo, which she can't play unless one of the aides helps her. Her mother's other favorite activity is the sing-along held every Tuesday and Thursday. Most days she doesn't even recognize Jill.

Jill's reaction to the situation, however, is very different from that of John. Sometimes Jill arrives during the Bingo game and sits beside her mother as she's playing. Instead of thinking how much her mother's mental capacity has declined, she notes that her mother has a smile on her face. Jill is so happy that there are still things her mother enjoys.

Although her mother usually doesn't recognize her, it's obvious that she enjoys Jill's visits. As far as the diapers her mother wears, Jill isn't upset by them. All babies wear them and that isn't depressing to anyone.

To a great extent, our attitudes about long-term care facilities and people with dementia influence how we view them. We must look at the roses and let the thorns pass into the background.

If we are in denial and try to insist that our loved one talk and behave like a 'normal' person, we will be miserable every time we see the person. If we focus on what our loved one *can't* do rather than what he or she still *can* do, visiting will be painful. If we focus on the thorns instead of the roses our distress will know no end.

Dear Lord, When I reach my darkest moments, help me to see the roses rather than the thorns surrounding my loved one. Amen.

Marie Marley, PhD (Interdenominational)

REAPING THE HARVEST

So let us not become weary in doing good, for at the proper time we will reap a harvest if we do not give up. - Galatians 6:9 (NIV)

Jean was one of the ladies with Alzheimer's I volunteered to visit every week. When I first met her she was wheelchair-bound and talked very little or not at all. I immediately set about finding a way to connect with her. Hopefully, to add some meaning to her life.

One day I showed her a book of colorful flowers but she didn't seem to really enjoy it. So then I tried having conversations with her. She sat mostly in silence, saying only a word or two from time to time and occasionally nodding her head in agreement.

So the next time I went I took my CD player and played some Mozart for her. Music can often reach people with Alzheimer's on a level we cannot. But that didn't seem to be effective either.

Finally I decided the best thing to do would be to simply sit near her, hold her hand and talk to her without expecting any response. Week after week I sat beside Jean, held her weak, tiny hand, and talked to her softly.

I didn't expect a response and I didn't get one. I had no idea what she was thinking or feeling. I didn't know if she was even aware of my presence. But I kept on keeping on, kept on holding her hand and talking to her as the weeks went by.

Then one day during my weekly visit I was surprised and overcome with emotion. As I was holding her hand she slowly reached over with her other hand and placed it on my arm ever so gently. Then she looked deeply into my eyes and began caressing my arm.

That was when I knew she'd been aware of my presence. It's when I knew that I'd made a connection with her after all. That she'd felt my affection. It's when I knew she'd been touched by it. And that I'd made a difference in her life.

When I went to visit the following week Jean wasn't in her room. I asked an aide where she was and was told to go and talk to the program director. I couldn't imagine why.

"I'm really sorry to have to tell you this, Marie," Melissa said. "But Jean passed away yesterday." I was struck with sadness, but took a little consolation in the knowledge that I hadn't given up.

Dear Lord, please give me the strength and patience to keep on keeping on when things seem hopeless, that I might one day make a difference in the life of a person with Alzheimer's. Amen.

Marie Marley, PhD (Interdenominational)

BEYOND THE WHY?

Read Psalm 22 & Psalm 23

The words are well known and so heart felt, "My God, My God Why Have You Forsaken Me?" Jesus' words on the cross are still being said by those living with the hope-crushing experience of Alzheimer's disease. As caregivers we will hold the hands; our shoulder will be cried on, we will sit by the bedside and our understanding of a loving God will be challenged. In my 30 years of ministry I have often joined those who are hurting in reading the 22nd Psalm; asking God the question, "Why?" We sometimes need to hear permission from clergy to speak our mind to God; additionally the validation of finding our feelings spoken in scripture and by Christ himself can be freeing. When everyone you know, plus hundreds you don't know are praying and the disease continues to progress, isn't it natural to ask where God is? We inevitably are confronted by the fact that bad things happen to good people and one of the important lessons we need to learn is that life is not fair!

I suspect that there was some spiritual wisdom involved in the placement of these two psalms next to each other. The epiphany ("Aha" moment) comes when we see beyond our feeling abandoned to discover that our hope is not in the fairness of life; rather, our hope is in the faithfulness of God's love for us.

I became a chaplain because, as a student, I met older women with cancer who could tell me a long list of the horrible things that had occurred in their lives, ending the conversation with, "And you know, Pastor, through it all God has been good." These women bore witness that the Jesus on the cross is not a sign of our distance from God; rather, God has made the cross a sign of God's bridging the gap in order to stand in solidarity with each of us. The cross is the sign that, regardless of what life may hand us, nothing can separate us from the love of God. God is our Shepherd, and even when we walk through the valley of the shadow of death we need fear no evil.

Lord God, You have called Your servants to ventures of which we cannot see the ending, by paths as yet untrodden, through perils unknown. Give us faith to go out with good courage, not knowing where we go; only that Your hand is leading us and Your love supporting us; through Jesus Christ our Lord. Amen.

Rev. Brian McCaffrey (Evangelical Lutheran Church in America)

SEARCHING FOR SILENCE

In the morning, while it was still very dark, he got up and went out to a deserted place, and there he prayed. - Mark 1:35

Recently, I spent a couple of days at a worship conference that was mostly focused on tapping into the contemplative life. I am attracted to the goal of living a life in union with God, but rarely achieve success.

Henry Nouwen wrote in his wonderful short reflection on Christian Leadership, *In the Name of Jesus*, "the loud, boisterous noises of the world make us deaf to the soft, gentle, and loving voice of God."

Noise is a great barrier to the contemplative life. Noise from without and noise from within.

I have worked to limit the noise from without by limiting technology use in my home and choosing to spend driving time in silence when possible. But many times I'm thwarted by the noise from within in my goal of contemplation: the cacophony of I-need-to-remember-to-do and how-will-I-ever-get-to-that.

If we expect and hope to hear the still, small voice of Christ leading us, how could we ever expect to hear it in the midst of the boisterous noise that Henry Nouwen describes?

Caregivers are deluged with a multitude of concerns, "boisterous noises," in the 36-hour day that is the reality of their experience. Yet, even in the frenetic busyness of caregiving, God can be present. Brother Lawrence and Saint Francis experienced the presence of God in mundane activities such as washing pots or feeding animals.

Early in the morning, Jesus went to a quiet place outside of the noise and bustle to pray. We can take our cue from Christ. The contemplative life that leads to union with Christ begins with a reduction in noise and a searching for silence.

Word of God, speak.

Father, lead us to the quiet place to meet You. Help us to find rest for our souls. We find our center and our peace in Your presence. Amen.

Hunter Mobley, Executive Pastor, Christ Church, Nashville (Christian)

WAITING AND IN-BETWEEN

... But those who wait for the Lord shall renew their strength. - Isaiah 40:31

Each year after Pentecost we enter a new season in the Christian calendar, Ordinary Time, that comes between, after and before the great celebration seasons of the church.

What's with all the waiting? The celebration passes so quickly and the seasons of in-between-ness last so long.

And isn't this the way of our lives as well? The celebrations seem few and far between and from celebration to celebration, we wait for something great, something transcendent. We wait to escape the ordinariness of time—the regularness of life. If we're not careful, we spend our whole lives waiting. Wishing away the days. Longing for the parades.

And the time between the demands of caring for a person with dementia in the present and the dread of what may eventually occur only exacerbates the burden of caregiving.

But God, in spite of our wanderlust for celebration, has ordered our calendar and our lives with long and always recurring seasons of ordinariness, regularness and waiting. He meant for it to be this way. Celebrations bring temporary joy. But the joy that comes in waiting and in regular times is abiding. The waiting, in-between seasons. These are the times when we can find the deepest and most abiding joy. And we find it from pressing deeper into our hearts, into devotion to God, and into our communities. These are the regular things that fill our ordinary times with great joy if we wait with intention.

The early morning cup of coffee and prayer may be the time that God decides to visit us. The Thursday night family dinner could be the moment when intimacy with our spouse builds to a new level of joy. The long conversation with a friend at work may reveal to us that we really aren't alone after all. The new book on the nightstand can ignite our imagination. The long drive into the country may lead to a vista of beauty that reminds us that God is truly present and working. And the thunderstorm might lead us to thank God that he is bigger and grander than anything that we could ever hope for or imagine.

Life is mostly filled with waiting and in-between times. And we get to choose the intention that we bring to these times. We can wish them away and find joy in the five or six days of the year when we join the parade. Or we can find joy in every season. Deep, abiding and lasting joy. The joy that is found in waiting with intention.

Father, help us to wait well. Help us to wait with intention. To enjoy every day and every moment. Help us to be present in each moment. Amen.

Hunter Mobley, Executive Pastor, Christ Church, Nashville (Christian)

THE POWER OF COMPASSION

May I be filled with lovingkindness. May I be safe. May I be well.
May I be at ease and happy. May you be filled with lovingkindness.
May you be safe. May you be well. May you be at ease and happy.
- adapted from Buddhist monk Jack Kornfields's Lovingkindness Meditation

As a caregiver for my mother, I have struggled with knowing if my ways of caring for her were right or good. I always want to do and be better, and to always be there for her. Yet I also have my own life, my husband and son, and often feel shame at not being able to be everything for my mom. Times like this are hard for a caregiver to manage, and we can fall into judging ourselves harshly. I often forget to have compassion for myself, and how hard not only is the act of caregiving, but also how hard it is to watch my loved one change and seem so far away from me.

While I want to be the best caregiver I can be, I also sometimes have a difficult time coping with how Mom's dementia affects her. Sometimes she acts differently; and negative personality traits come out; the sheer time of caregiving is overwhelming and I wish she were easier to care for. In those times, I am too reactive. I realize that in my struggle, I forget to have compassion for her and what this illness is doing to her.

Having compassion and understanding for ourselves and other people is difficult. It takes practice because life is hard; and, when we are overwhelmed, we can stop living in that place of compassion and, instead, start reacting from a place of fear. In order to cultivate compassion, I repeat the meditation above, while holding my mother and me in my heart. Compassion heals the soul. It lessens reactivity, and gives us a chance to pause and reach into our souls in order to act with compassion and love.

Spirit of Life and Love, in times when I struggle to understand my loved one with dementia, may I take pause and let compassion guide me. Compassion reminds me to be kind to myself when I'm frustrated and afraid, and allows me to be less reactive and more understanding to others. May the Spirit of Love and Compassion guide us as caregivers in this journey through dementia. Amen.

Rev. Katie Norris (Unitarian Universalist)

MAMA'S RED SHOES

My health may fail, and my spirit may grow weak, but God remains the strength of my heart; he is mine forever. - Psalm 73:26 (NLT)

I stand silently staring at the rack of shoes in the bottom of my mom's closet. The revelation comes to me that these shoes, composed of many colors and styles, represent my mom's personality. Some sparkle with rhinestones while others reflect well-worn edges. I am saddened to think that my mom will never wear these shoes again as she lies in a bed, ravaged by a stroke and dementia.

We now paint her toes in many of the bright colors that once adorned her feet as sandals or "Sunday" shoes. Mama laughs as I enter her room at the nursing home. She eagerly tells me that she has spent the day driving her red convertible. I smile and say, "Well, it was certainly a great day for a drive." She launches into a beautiful story of a road long-since paved. Mama describes what she is wearing, including her red shoes with the rhinestones.

Deciding to share these shoes with those who can wear them is the "right thing to do," I reason, but my heart longs for the days when the red leather shoes adorned my mom's feet as she walked into church.

I tuck the red shoes in my bag for a safe, special place in my own closet.

Our Father, Your love is our refuge as hearts ache for a moment of "knowing" in a loved one's eyes. Give us strength to appreciate and celebrate the time we have together with our loved ones lost in the sea of dementia. Amen.

Laura Pannell, PhD, CPG (United Methodist)

A VALUABLE LESSON

We are not human beings having a spiritual experience. We are spiritual beings having a human experience. - Pierre Telhiard de Chardin, The Phenomenon of Man, 1955

There is a theory that claims that we are all only six degrees of separation apart from anyone else. We welcome this theory because we live in an elaborate system of separation, which we have accepted as true. Now we feel good to think that we are only six steps away from all other people. Why does this make us feel better?

Because we believe in separation when in fact there is no separation. Life is ultimately connected at all times. Whatever separation we feel and whatever barriers we perceive are made up of our own creations. Reality lies not in what we have created, but in what God has created. Life and connectedness are the only reality, and we will find this to be true when we look for ways in which life is connected. If we can imagine going beyond what society tells us are the impairments that come with dementia, we will discover new possibilities. We will find connectedness and joy. It is possible to have a rich and wonderful relationship with people living with dementia.

Several years ago my mother faced one of her biggest challenges and embarked on one of her most important triumphs when she was diagnosed with dementia. Her triumph was that of the spirit, because she continued to be who she was. She always taught us that it isn't what you do but who you are that matters. While she was affected physically she was unaffected spiritually. Her human experience changed but the essence of her being remained the same. It was a celebration of joy every time I was in her presence and this continued to be true while we all prepared for her transition.

One night one of her nurses came in, looked at her and said, "She is a class act right up until the end." Another commented that Mom was going to be teaching us how to "get it right" even as she passed away. And that is what she did.

My mother was, and still is, a beautiful spirit that touched many lives and taught me my most important lessons. She taught me that our spirit transcends everything, because it is the essence of life, and the bond of our spirit is as strong as it has ever been. Thank you, Mom, for teaching me my most valuable lesson.

O God of grace, help us to see the spirit of life that You have given us. Guide us as we celebrate the lives of those living with dementia and help us continue to be witnesses to their life, whole and beautiful just as You have created them to be. Amen and Amen. Let it be.

Rev. Linn Possell (The United Church of Christ)

THE WOMEN WHO CARE

Meanwhile, standing near the cross of Jesus were his mother, and his mother's sister, Mary the wife of Clopas, and Mary Magdalene. - John 19:25

My father, in the last stages of Alzheimer's disease, had not spoken a sentence in some time. Beset by pneumonia, "the old person's friend," Dad spent the final weeks leading up to the end transitioning from nursing home to hospital, then eventually to an inpatient hospice facility for his final earthly days.

In what I have come to think of as a "drawing in," Dad's physical presence in our world became enwrapped increasingly in a quilt of those who cared, and for whom he had cared for so long. Pulled ever more closely toward this one who had been our rock and dearest friend, something deep inside us knew we must come together and share in the great mystery of death and departing that we sensed was imminent. It was to be a precious, sacred time.

The hospice days and nights were filled with singing, praying, hand-holding and reminiscing around the bedside. The one who had not spoken in weeks mouthed words of old hymns that had shaped his early faith, the anchor that held fast in dementia's turbulent sea.

In that final night, Dad's wandering gaze drew, laser-like, to focus on the corner of the ceiling, and remained there for hours. To the others, I questioned why he might be staring there.

Finally, I asked, "Papa, what are you looking at?"

In a flash of cloud-piercing clarity, he turned his eyes to me and said, "Mama."

The others left, and for the next few hours my Mother and I, each kneeling by the bedside, cried, prayed, and shared all our strength to help him Home. He breathed his last breath at 4:10 am, September 15, 2007. And I believe his mother was there to help him, too.

Strong. Self-giving. Nurturing. Faithful even in death's dark valley were the women who cared.

Almighty yet ever-nurturing God, thank you for the women who care, who embody what surely represents the sacred feminine within the Divine heart. Amen.

Daniel C. Potts, MD, FAAN, Elder (Presbyterian Church, USA)

THE GIFT

Read Genesis 22:1-14

So Abraham called that place, "The Lord Will Provide." And to this day it is said, "On the mountain of the Lord it will be provided." - Genesis 22:14 (NIV)

From the unenlightened state in which I found myself as a supplementary caregiver for my father, Lester E. Potts, Jr., I saw a broken man, a murky reflection of the one I had known and loved.

When he entered Caring Days, a dementia daycare center started by our church, Dad had stopped smiling, couldn't speak in complete sentences, and had lost the utilitarian ingenuity that had characterized his entire life. Dad could fix anything. But no longer. Even those once-capable hands seemed lost and confused.

At Caring Days, Dad was honored for being no more and no less than he was in each moment of his existence. He was validated and affirmed as a person with relational gifts, as someone who had something to give to the world. Affliction could not steal this gift. In fact, *its impact was made greater through the suffering state of the giver.*

The gift was art. Beautiful, vibrant, expressive watercolors from the one who had never painted prior to onset of the disease. This miraculous unfolding of Dad's heart through creativity infused a tincture of hope into the lives of those who cared for him. We stood dumbfounded, and so very grateful.

In his book, *The Gift: Creativity and the Artist in the Modern World,* Lewis Hyde writes "The gift that is not used will be lost, while the one that is passed along will be abundant." We have experienced this through Dad's art. The staff at Caring Days believed in him, shared their gifts, and listened with their spirits for his song. Dad added his true voice, and we joined in the singing. But it was God who provided the tune amidst the suffering silence of Alzheimer's.

The very nature of the gift is that it must be shared, as it has been shared with us.

God, as we walk with our loved ones up the barren mountain of dementia, help us to know that You will provide the gifts that will carry us through, enabling us to be faithful and compassionate caregivers every step of the way. Help us to always be willing to share our gifts. Amen.

Daniel C. Potts, MD, FAAN, Elder (Presbyterian Church, USA)

LETTING GO

"When we establish within our thought a nonresistance to that Power which is greater than we are, we are at the same time accepting within ourselves a stability that is the stability of the universe. We find ourselves secure, for we know that we are part of That which causes change but is never affected by any of the changes." - Ernest Holmes, Science of Mind Magazine, January 2001

When I worked as a hospice chaplain, I met with families going through many challenges with their loved ones in the process of transition. One family had a beautiful way to be with their mother in the last stages of Alzheimer's. They sat in her room and sang to her. The songs awoke something in her that allowed her to connect, albeit with a distant glimmer. They had come to terms with their mother's situation, and were letting go with love. The singing gave everyone comfort, and most assuredly would remain in their memories after her passing.

I had another client—a son who was caring for his mother in her final days. Even though eating was difficult for her, he gave her a probiotic diet, wanting her to drink concoctions he made for her, and generally fed her very healthy but unappetizing food. He told me that she really liked ice cream, but he didn't want her to have it because it wasn't good for her. He wanted to make her better. Clearly he had not come to terms with where she was on her journey, even though hospice was now making daily visits to her home. Our hospice team assured him that at this point, she deserved to have the food she enjoyed over the food that might be healthier. After that, she got her ice cream.

Alzheimer's seems to rob us of the person we knew. It feels cruel. As the first signs show up in our loved one, we can delude ourselves into thinking it's a temporary lapse and they will bounce back and be okay. Slowly, gradually, we recognize that there is a decline taking place. This is hard to accept for our loved one and for us. Resisting the changes only causes more pain and discomfort. Acceptance allows us to move forward, rather than cling to what was.

Accepting what *is* allows us to surrender. As we witness the changes and the slow farewell, we realize that our love does not diminish. Often it deepens. Our life circumstance may change, but the love of God never changes. As we surrender, and let the Spirit move in our life, we find ways to cope with what is. Letting go clears a space for greater good to enter.

Byars and Beckwith say it well in their song: *I release and I let go, I let the Spirit run my life; And my heart is open wide, yes, I'm only here for God; No more struggle, no more strife, with my faith I see the light; I am free in the Spirit, yes, I'm only here for God.*

I surrender to the One Power that is greater than I am. As I do, I am given the wisdom and the courage to walk through the challenges I face with an open heart. Divine Love never changes—and the love I felt for my loved one is just as real as it ever was—even though my loved one has changed. As I let go, I find peace.

Rev. Dr. Peggy Price, Center for Spiritual Living (Interdenominational)

ENOUGH

Let me sing for my beloved my love-song concerning his vineyard: My beloved had a vineyard... He dug it and cleared it of stones, and planted it with choice vines; he built a watch-tower... and hewed out a wine vat in it; he expected it to yield grapes, but it yielded wild grapes. And now... judge between me and my vineyard. What more was there to do for my vineyard that I have not done...? When I expected it to yield grapes, why did it yield wild grapes? - Isaiah 5:1-4

Dag Hammarskjöld, Secretary-General of the United Nations (1953-61) kept record of, as he put it, "negotiations" with himself and God. After his untimely death in a plane crash in 1961, the diary was published, with the English translation titled *Markings*. This remarkable volume is amply rewarding to anyone who reflects upon these simple yet profound thoughts. One of the most meaningful for me regarding caregiving is this admonition: "Do what you can—and the task will rest lightly in your hand, so lightly that you will be able to look forward to the more difficult tests which may be awaiting you."

I wish caregivers could hear and accept that advice. It seems that often they spend much time and energy wishing to have a "do-over" of some interaction so that they could try harder, get less angry, and do a "little better job." Indeed, many people expend so much energy fretting about having done what they perceive as an inadequate job that they become almost immobilized as far as living in the present is concerned.

I am not saying that we should ever do less than our very best on any task that comes to us—the higher we set our ideals the higher we are apt to get, even if we don't reach them. But I am advocating the approach Hammarskjöld suggests: Do what you can with what you have to work with; accept the outcome of your best effort; and then get on with those "more difficult tests which may be awaiting you."

Good scriptural warrant is available for this attitude: In Isaiah 5, the prophet sings a song using images of a vineyard for Israel and the keeper for God. In verse 4, God—the omnipotent Creator, the One who should be able to get the exact results the Keeper wants—almighty God asks, "What more was there to do for my vineyard that I have not done in it? When I expected it to yield grapes, why did it yield wild grapes?" If even *God* sometimes accepts less than the ideal results desired from God's own actions, surely we can do what we can and trust God with the results.

God, help us to do our best in all caregiving tasks, and grant us grace to accept the outcome, trusting You to use the results for Your loving purposes. Amen.

The Reverend Stephen Sapp, PhD (Presbyterian Church, USA)

WHAT DO YOU DO?

"The kind of work God usually calls you to is the kind of work that you need most to do and that the world most needs to have done..." - Frederick Buechner, Wishful Thinking

My friend Charles was CEO of a multinational corporation. He had literally thousands of employees and he loved the business world—visioning, making decisions, managing people, solving problems. He was exceptionally good at it, successful and happy in his work but he took early retirement to care for his wife who had Alzheimer's. She died recently and, after 20 years, he is facing the BIG question of old age: Who am I, now that I am not a caregiver?

I was a caregiver, too, for many years, and I am asking the same question. So are Charlotte and Barbara and Susan, recent widows, with whom I talk often. All of us have spent the last decade or more caring for our husbands, at home and/or in a care facility. It was probably the most important work we will ever do. We had a mission, a purpose. And, without that sense of calling, we feel a bit lost. What now?

Can a brilliant and talented CEO find satisfaction in delivering Meals on Wheels?

Will a woman who once was actively involved in many community organizations and president of the church council be content to pour coffee and clean up after the worship service?

How could an 84-year old volunteer be matched to an appropriate need?

The trouble is, we are not willing to settle. We have so little time left that we want to use it well. We feel an urgency to make a contribution to society that somehow, in some manner, seems as important as what we have done in the past. And yet...we don't want the long hours, the interruptions and the demands of jobs we had when we were younger.

In fact, we are not looking for a job! Even in old age (or maybe especially now) we want a vocation. We want to find ourselves again, we are looking for answers. But for awhile, we all have to live with the questions. John O'Donohue describes our state in this excerpt from his prayer, "For Suffering":

You have been forced to enter empty time. The desire that drove you has relinquished. There is nothing else to do now but rest and patiently learn to receive the self. You have forsaken in the race of days. Amen.

Anne Simpson (The United Church of Christ)

FACING THE DOUBTS AND DILEMMAS

When things are going well for you, be glad, and when trouble comes, just re-member: God sends both happiness and trouble: you never know what is going to happen next. - Ecclesiastes 7:14 (Good News Bible: Catholic Study Edition)

My mother is now a resident in an Alzheimer's unit and is in capable hands. Now I need to determine how I will function in my new role as a post-placement caregiver. At first I would cringe when asked how my mother was doing. When I told them about the placement issue, they would respond, "Oh, you put your mother in a nursing home!" I soon realized that many people don't understand how the quality of residential care has changed recently. Hearing their responses, I realized that I didn't want to be judged and that I needed to learn how to address the social stigma implied in their responses.

In the past I thought I could overcome the challenges I faced; I was "in control." Now, however, though I'm aware I have not abandoned my mother, I want others to know I am still her caregiver. This role doesn't stop at the door of the nursing home. I realized I was becoming mired in guilt and kept asking myself if I had made the wrong decision.

At first, I didn't know how to act. Would it be necessary to become a "helicopter"-type post-placement caregiver? Would I need to hover over every aspect of my mother's care, or should I place my trust in the professional caregivers while continuing to love and care for her in a different capacity? Frightened, I tried to focus on the positives.

I want to be a compassionate, positive caregiver who is watchful and engaged with my mother while dealing with my own fears and doubts as best I can. She will always be my mother; and, I will do my best to help her new caregivers know who she still is, though Alzheimer's has up-ended her life. I don't want them to see her as an "empty shell." I need to keep her spirit intact and alive during these trying times.

I am extremely thankful for the compassionate professional caregivers who have kept my mother safe and as comfortable as possible. Learning to let go of the "helicopter" mentality, I now take time to enjoy the blessings of life. When the end comes, I will hold my head high and be grateful that I did my best. I will know that all is well and my mother's spirit is free!

Lord, as I awake each morning, I ask for the strength to deal with the ups and the downs of life. I pray for the assurance that I am doing my best and will continue with the resolve to be the best caregiver my dearest loved one needs. As long as my loved one lives, help me to care compassionately. Help me always to understand that the journey we are taking will continue into eternity. Amen.

Barbara Stephens (Roman Catholic)

A PRESENCE IN THE STORM

That day when evening came, he said to his disciples, "Let us go over to the other side." Leaving the crowd behind, they took him along, just as he was, in the boat. There were also other boats with him. A furious squall came up, and the waves broke over the boat, so that it was nearly swamped. Jesus was in the stern, sleeping on a cushion. The disciples woke him and said to him, "Teacher, don't you care if we drown?" He got up, rebuked the wind and said to the waves, "Quiet! Be still!" Then the wind died down and it was completely calm. - Mark 4:37-39 (NIV)

My wife gets irritated with me when severe weather blows. I am slow to move, being the last to the basement and only then after much cajoling. I hasten to say though, with her help I have gained a healthy respect for storms, and when necessary, will take precautions. But I can sleep through a gale. The reason behind this goes back to a childhood experience and has also come to be one of the primary ways in which I understand God's Holy Presence.

One night, when I was four years old, a storm began to brew. The sound of the wind howling around the eaves and shrubbery brushing against the house scared me. Hearing my cry, my father came to get in bed with me, cradling me in his arms. When the wind howled, he mimicked the sound in my ear. He scratched the sheet with his fingernails imitating the sound of the bushes scraping against the house from the force of the wind. Enveloped in his strong embrace, I fell fast asleep. He didn't make the storm go away, but his presence calmed the tempest in my heart.

I have often thought that perhaps the storm Jesus calmed was not so much the one on the sea as the storm in the disciples' hearts. These were seamen who had weathered storms before. Yet, they were nearly drowning. In their fear they cried out to Jesus who quieted the storm. Soothed by the Son of God, the disciples were able to draw upon their self-possessed skills to ride the seas and navigate their course to the other side.

Sometimes the demands of caring for a loved one break over you like billowing waves and it seems as though you are sinking. Yet, God is already in the flood with you. Assured by your faith and experience of the presence of your loving Father, your mind can be clear and your hands confident to take on the trials of the tasks at hand. As my dad embraced the fear of a scared little boy and as Jesus rose to calm the fear of the wind and the waves, even so, Abba, our Heavenly Father, knows our self-doubt, hears our cry and calms our weary hearts.

Dear God, in the midst of this stormy day, help me to remember that the grace of Your steadfast presence that has been sufficient to see me through prior storms, will be sufficient to help me weather even these challenges that toss me to and fro. May the comfort of Your strong embrace calm my weary heart. In the name of him who is the master of the wind and waves I pray. Amen.

Rev. Alan Swindall, LMFT (United Methodist)

ECCLESIASTES 3:1-8 FOR CAREGIVERS

by Richard L. Morgan and Jane Marie Thibault (© 2008)

There is a time for everything,

And a season for every activity under the heavens.

    a time to love the person and a time to hate the disease,

    a time to speak and a time to be silent,

    a time to be angry and a time to reconcile,

    a time to feel guilty and a time to forgive yourself,

    a time to cry a little and a time to laugh a lot,

    a time to welcome others and a time to be alone,

    a time to accept another treatment and a time to forgo more treatment,

    a time to ask for help and a time to act by oneself.

    a time for my loved one and a time for myself,

    a time to enjoy remembering and a time to embrace the present,

    a time to do more than is expected and a time to say 'good enough is good enough,'

    a time to care at home and a time for placement,

    a time to hold on to life and time to let go in death,

    a time to mourn and a time to move on.

PAINTED BITS OF BARK AND STONE AND TIN

"Grow old along with me! The best is yet to be, the last of life, for which the first was made. Our times are in His hand who saith, 'A whole I planned, youth shows but half; Trust God: see all, nor be afraid.'" - Robert Browning (1812-1889)

She won my heart in college when she lived across the street.
Her roommate was a friend of mine, who thought that we should meet.
I liked her looks and kindness, but what made our love begin
Was her painted bits of bark and stone and tin.

I'd leave for class each morning and come back again at dark
To find she'd left a love note, painted on a piece of bark,
Or maybe on a shiny rock, I'd spot as I walked in
Her painted bits of bark and stone and tin.

She'd stop and chat on campus when I'd study 'neath a tree,
And when she'd leave I'd open up my book again to see
A sweet verse on a rusted tin can lid she'd slipped within:
More painted bits of bark and stone and tin.

"Grow old along with me," she wrote, "the best is yet to be."
That Browning poem that she'd quote proved true for her and me.
Who'd guess that such a little rhyme would lifetime love begin
From painted bits of bark and stone and tin.

We married, raised two sons, and shared together forty years.
But now her health is slipping fast, the end of her life nears.
So it's my turn to care for her and keep love flowing in,
Bring her painted bits of bark and stone and tin.

I know that I must let her go, release her from my heart;
Let Present stop our Past, so our Forever love can start.
But I'd give all I treasure for that pleasure once again,
Of her painted bits of bark and stone and tin.
I'll let our Now end up our Then, our Always to begin,
Clutching painted bits of bark and stone and tin.

Don Wendorf, Psy.D. (Spiritual)

Reprinted with permission from Dr. Don Wendorf, Psy.D, *Caregiver Carols: A Musical, Emotional Memoir* (CreateSpace, May 2014).

FALL

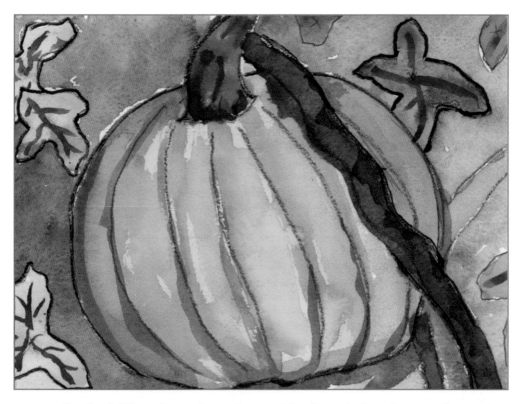

For our family, fall has always brought a quickening wind to the ever-shortening, bright blue days of the season. With the chill and swirling leaves came also a hint of mischief, and Dad always enjoyed playing a trick or two on the youth of our neighborhood. His pumpkin painting from middle stage Alzheimer's disease reminds me of the fun he had while attending Caring Days, the adult day center where his artistic talent was discovered. An annual Halloween Party brought a special opportunity to dress up and live in the moment, making the most of the season's changing colors. It also reminds us of the importance of laughter and play, and the childlike joy that can be found even on dark days.

A SPOUSE TRIES TO SUPPORT A CAREGIVER

Be joyful in hope, patient in affliction, faithful in prayer. - Romans 12:12 (NIV)

In the last few years my mother-in-law, Elizabeth, who is now 93, has progressed into an ever-deepening state of dementia. Out of necessity for her increasing physical frailty, she has gone from living with us to a senior apartment, then to a personal care home, and lastly to a nursing home. The nursing home provides excellent daily care, but since it is at some distance from us, my wife, Mary, can only manage to visit two or three times per week.

The visits always place an emotional toll on Mary. Elizabeth's attitude can range from somewhat pleasant to completely exasperating. Mary usually comes home exhausted and often full of guilt that she can't stop the negative attitude or the worsening memory problems of her mother. These emotions often carry over to the days she does not visit, so it provides an ever-present concern. When I accompany Mary on these visits, I understand her exasperation. However, I often fail to maintain that understanding after ending the visit, and I, too, feel guilty for not being more supportive.

Our lives have changed quite a bit since we first faced this challenge. There is much less time for us to share conversations and experiences with each other. As a spouse of a person caring for a parent with dementia, I confess that sometimes I am resentful of the time it takes from our lives together. I know I don't always listen attentively as she gives the details of her visits or the frequent care decisions she has to make. I find myself trying to cope with the emotional turmoil she endures by remaining detached rather than sharing her emotions. I pray that I will be more supportive, more understanding, and more patient with Mary as she continues to care for her mother.

Gracious God, help us to support our spouses or siblings as they provide their special love and care to parents living with dementia. Help us to maintain our compassion for the afflicted. Amen.

Gerald Cumer (Presbyterian, USA)

THE MEMORY CAFÉ: AN ISLE OF ACCEPTANCE

We do not want you to be uninformed, brothers and sisters, about the troubles we experienced in the province of Asia. We were under great pressure, far beyond our ability to endure, so that we despaired of life itself. Indeed, we felt we had received the sentence of death. But this happened that we might not rely on ourselves but on God, who raises the dead. - 2 Corinthians 1:8,9

We are social beings; seeking acceptance and trusted relationships. Yet, age and disabilities may confine and limit our social interactions to a few close friends and family members. Older persons with dementia may become isolated because friends and associates become confused by changes in their behavior. Names and facts may be lost with dementia, and this loss of memory can be unsettling. Devoted caregivers also may become isolated by the demands of meeting the needs of their loved one. Sometimes activities outside the home become a burden, and the pleasure associated with being accepted, with belonging to a group is unfulfilled.

The Memory Café was developed so that those with memory loss and those who love them might belong again. Families are welcomed, accepted, and respected when they arrive at the Café with an attitude that embraces and supports them wherever they are in the disease process. There are no unrealistic expectations as Café visitors share food and stories, experience art, and move to the music. Caregivers have experienced the losses of the disease and are not shocked by the behaviors of other Café guests, nor do they need explanation about the stresses that dominate the days of other caregivers. Memories of carefree moments from the past surface. Sometimes such memories are shared in words, sometimes not. The past matters little as the new connections and shared compassion offer the healing needed to move on to deal with the next day.

We cannot see within the minds of the families as they spend time together at the Café. We can only see the smiles, the reluctant departures and the warm hellos and farewells. Perhaps, most important, we see many of the same faces return month after month. Have we brought a glimmer of hope into the lives of these families? Have caregivers felt love and joy from their interactions if only for a brief moment? We cannot say with certainty, but we know that for an afternoon the clouds are parted, and we share a journey.

Our Heavenly Father, give us the courage and strength to support one another through this devastating illness. Help us to continue to show our love and compassion to those who are sick and those who love them so that they do not feel alone and isolated. Give us time for acceptance, reflection, and prayer so that hope is not lost. Amen.

Deborah D. Danner, PhD (Baptist)

THE TEACHER

An intelligent heart acquires knowledge, and the ear of the wise seeks knowledge.
- Proverbs 18:15 (ESV)

I thought I was going to offer spiritual support to Vickie. She had been showing increasingly significant signs of confusion and memory loss from Alzheimer's disease. But this day was different.

Vickie was not in her room, where I usually found her, but in the lounge, sitting at a table and talking with several other residents. There was one chair open, and I asked if I could join them. "Sure," said Vickie. I pulled up a chair, and soon realized that there was something important—something very good—happening at that table.

One resident was expressing her fears to Vickie. She said, "I just don't know what is going to happen to me tonight. I'm far from my home, and I don't know where I am going to sleep tonight." She was anxious and afraid, and crying out for help. I was ready to reassure her, but before I spoke, Vickie said to her, "Don't worry, I'll make sure you are safe tonight. You can come to my room, and sleep in my bed. I will sleep on the sofa, so I will be right next to you all night long. If you wake up and are scared, just look over at me, and I will be there watching over you. I'll wave to you to let you know that everything is alright."

Vickie's words worked like a healing balm, and her friend became calm and was able to put her fears aside. Just then, another resident who was sitting at the table, who is not able to speak, turned his wheelchair around and left the table, heading for his room.

Vickie got up and went over to him. "Stan," she said, "Even though you weren't talking, I want you to know that we enjoyed having you with us. You are an important part of the group. Please come back any time and join us."

I was stunned: a woman who was locked in combat with Alzheimer's, often in confusion and distress herself, was reaching out with seasoned wisdom and compassion to those around her.

Vickie taught me that day, by example, how to conduct myself as a hospice chaplain: she was focused not on herself, but on the needs of those around her. She brought love, reassurance and the healing touch of Christ to her neighbors.

Thank you, Lord, for good teachers. May I be open each day to learn from the wisdom acquired by Your people in every walk of life. Amen.

Chaplain Drew DeCrease (Roman Catholic Deacon)

FINE. I'M FINE!

God is faithful, and he will not let you be tested beyond your strength, but with the testing he will also provide the way out so that you may be able to endure it.
- 1 Corinthians 10:13

People quote this scripture a lot, and maybe we think it is helpful to tell folks who are completely overwhelmed that "God won't give you more than you can handle." Worse, we implicitly or explicitly tag on a good old-fashioned Americanized pull-yourself-up-by-your-bootstraps clause that leaves everyone feeling alone and alienated from God. "God won't give you more than you can handle *on your own.*"

It is okay to say that you are not fine when you are overwhelmed as a caregiver. Not even St. Paul, that bundle of courage, self-denial, and Holy Spirit energy would advise you to take on a challenge of this size "on your own." He is writing to a whole church community (not just to you) and he is writing about keeping the faith. The actual scripture says that "you will not be tempted beyond what you can bear," and he means that you will not ever want to let go of your faith. He reminds the church of the history of the Israelites who came out of bondage in Egypt. In the terrifying, vast wilderness of their Exodus journey, they were tempted to feel lost and alone, but each time they called to God, God responded with protection and generosity.

Even in moments when you feel alone, know that God is with you. Stand firm in your faith.

God is present in the good company of your faith community. When they ask if you are fine, let them know that you are absolutely *not* doing a great job of bearing all of this "on your own." Let them be brothers and sisters to you. Let them in your home and your life, knowing that they will walk alongside you with words and actions of support, encouragement, and prayer.

Faith has never been a Do-It-Yourself proposition. We are meant to live faith out in love in the context of community.

Loving God, even in my most frustrating moments, I know that You are with me. You know when I am not fine. Nudge me to grasp the hands of help that are extended to me. I will know that this is You at work, and I will praise You. Amen.

Rev. Paige Eaves (United Methodist)

I LOVE YOU, TOO

"Our loves are only symbols of an unknown immortality.
Where communion is deep, there exists no separation at all,
for what needs telling those we love is understood already,
and what is supposed to be gone and past is often more real than ever."
- Cedric Wright, Words of the Earth, 1960

We caregivers often berate ourselves for the things that go unsaid.

There are many reasons and many of them unknown even to ourselves as to why we remain silent. In my own case, I thought that if I voiced my sorrow it would discourage my loved ones and swallow me up.

My first encounter with death was losing my mother when I was 27. Six years earlier, she had suffered a stroke which left her partially paralyzed. We never spoke of her illness, but held on to a false optimism that she would improve and get well. Twenty-eight years later, as my dad lay dying, I was better at expressing my love and my loss, and at giving Dad permission to die.

But I remained strangely quiet throughout the 15 years of my husband's battle with dementia. Again, I didn't want to say anything that would discourage him and I didn't want him to see me grieving, even as we were losing every semblance of the life that we shared together. Miraculously, the day before he died, I understood that this was a gift I owed him. I knew that, while he could no longer understand my words, he would understand my love and that my tears, which were sure to flow, would not frighten him. And so I took his hands in mine and looked directly into his eyes and, as the tears fell, thanked him for the many gifts of his presence and his love in my life. He listened intently and, when I was through, spoke his last words to me, "I love you, too."

So, while I encourage you to share your thanksgivings and your goodbyes, please do not be too hard on yourself if you have not been able to do so. Love is expressed in so many ways; sometimes silently. Your loved ones know. And they would not want to see you grieving.

Heavenly Father, Give us the courage to speak our hearts to those we love. If, because of our nature, circumstances, or fear, we have not been able to do so, allow us to forgive ourselves and know that "what needs telling those we love is understood already." Amen.

Lynda Everman (United Methodist)

THE "PERFECT" DAUGHTER

Honor your father and your mother, so that your days may be long in the land that the Lord your God is giving you. - Exodus 20:12

Within the past six months, Mattie's life changed dramatically. Her son graduated from college; but, since he had no job or money, he needed to move back home. Three months ago, Mattie's daughter filed for divorce, and along with her four-year-old daughter, moved in with her parents. Mattie's husband was recently promoted at work and has spent more time on the road. And now Mattie's mother, who began showing signs of mild cognitive impairment about two years ago, has been diagnosed with Alzheimer's.

Until recently, Mattie believed that she lived the life of "a perfect daughter." Mattie and her mother often did things together. They went shopping, attended weekly worship services and church school, and vacationed together each summer. But now the world feels like it is closing in on her. Because of her mother's dementia, Mattie becomes easily agitated, frustrated and angered. Although she feels guilty about her attitude toward her mother, Mattie complains that she just never imagined that her mother would need so much help.

Lately, Mattie has been crying at night, embarrassed and ashamed at her behavior towards her mother. Although she has never physically struck her, Mattie has verbally attacked her mother and said some very mean things to her.

A few weeks ago following Sunday morning worship, Mattie confided in her pastor concerning her anger and lack of self-control in dealing with her mother's Alzheimer's disease. Her pastor was aware of an Alzheimer's support group that was meeting regularly at the local hospital. He suggested that Mattie attend. Later that week Mattie made contact with the support group leader and began participating regularly.

Learning more about Alzheimer's disease and having the opportunity to freely share with others in her support group concerning her fears, frustration, and guilt has had a very positive effect on Mattie's life. While she no longer sees herself as being "the perfect daughter," she now realizes that even with her mother's deteriorating cognitive functioning, Mattie's love for her mother has grown stronger and she is finding new ways of being a more loving and caring daughter. In reality, Mattie is becoming the "perfect" daughter for her mother.

O loving God, You know my desires and my weaknesses, my longings and my failures. Guide me in the path of peace and grant me wisdom to face the challenges that later life brings. Grant me the confidence, strength, and courage to honor my parents as they face the challenges and struggles of old age. Help me grow in my understanding that old age can be a blessing and not an adversity, a gift and not a curse. Amen.

Rev. Dr. Richard H. Gentzler, Jr. (United Methodist)

DOWNEASTER

And there arose a fierce gale of wind, and the waves were breaking over the boat so much that the boat was already filling up. Jesus Himself was in the stern, asleep on the cushion; and they woke Him and said to Him, "Teacher, do You not care that we are perishing?" And He got up and rebuked the wind and said to the sea, "Hush, be still." And the wind died down and it became perfectly calm. - Mark 4:37-39

Waves crash along the shore of an eroded beach; slowly his memories are becoming out of reach. And tomorrow is today, and today is yesterday.

But behind closed eyes, such a fantastic life, with no more color. Now his memories are only in black and white.

Storm clouds gather on the bay as the old boat captain readies his Downeaster to sail away. He lights a cigar and pours himself a glass of wine, and tries real hard to remember a better time.

Turning the ship's wheel, he heads into the storm, puts on his jacket; he's trying to keep warm. Lightning scatters across an unforgiving sky. Raindrops collect in the storm drain he calls life.

The old boat captain slowly turns his ship to face the wind. There's no marlin to be caught in rough seas like this. A voice full of prayer, broken rosaries, He's left in the hand of God and the monster out at sea.

"The storm's only gonna get worse from here." But he heads further into the storm "cause there's nothing left to fear."

He holds a picture of his wife close to his heart. He smiles and closes his eyes and thanks God for letting him come this far. Memories of his wife, his kids, have begun to fade. He comes to realize *tomorrow* is today.

The storm's now cleared; water's calm as glass. The old man and his vessel have found serenity at last.

I guess that old man kept true to what he did; He never stopped working; at least he never thought he did.

(In my lifetime I have seen the sadness and despair that dementia causes. Watching people suffer through this disease provided the inspiration for "Downeaster.")

Loving God, no matter how far we sail and how rough the seas, bring our souls to anchor in the 'haven of rest' that is the deep ocean of Your Divine Presence. Amen.

Joseph J. Gombita (Roman Catholic)

ANSWERING THE CALL

"O my dear son! Though it be but the weight of a grain of mustard-seed, and though it be in a rock, or in the heavens, or in the earth, God brings it forth. God is Subtle, Aware. O my dear son! Establish worship and enjoin kindness and forbid iniquity, and be patient; that is of the steadfast heart of things." - The Noble Quran, 31:16,17

I was a child when one of my mom's friends was diagnosed with dementia. She was so kind to me and I became so close to her that I asked my grandfather to consider her as a wife after being a widow for so long. Though he refused, I called her "Grandpa's wife" and it became her nickname. I spent so much time with her, talking and listening to her stories about her younger years, and learning her delicious recipes. I loved shopping with her, especially as she walked so fast and managed to put a smile on every person's face. Over time she began forgetting things like where she put her items; I would say to her, "You're getting old, 'Grandpa's wife!'" I just never imagined that one day she would forget me too.

It was a new experience for everyone, especially when she started forgetting us and becoming afraid of people! My mom rented an apartment for her that would allow her to secure herself in a home with a gated exterior. Unfortunately, people made fun of her and showed no compassion for such a feeble elderly woman in need of special care.

Her visits to us became less frequent and we were unable to communicate well with her. Mom hired a lady to stay with her and keep her company and attend to her needs.

One day, possibly the last time I saw her in our house, she was in a rush talking about people who wanted to invade her home and steal her belongings. She broke something and someone made a negative comment. My dad later shared the following story with me: A father was setting the table for dinner with his young son and started putting a plastic plate, cup and plastic utensils for one person at the table. The son asked, "Dad, I don't eat any more with plastic!" His father replied, "It is not for you, it is for Grandpa, as I don't want him to break the china!" So one day, when the father was shopping with his son, the son went to get some plastic plates, cups and utensils. The father asked, "Why did you get these?" The boy replied, "It is for you and mom when you grow old so that when I have my own expensive china, you will come and eat with me and my family!"

Dear Lord! Shower us and those around us who suffer from dementia with Your Mercy and Love so we can share it with them. Strengthen us with kindness and compassion so they can feel safe and secure when they see us. Grant us the ability to see and discern between their behaviors and their souls so we can bring them tranquility and joy in this difficult journey. And choose us from among all people to be the ones who answer Your call in serving them. Amen!

Maria Khani, Educator and Spiritual Counselor (Muslim)

GOD KNOWS ME, EVEN WHEN YOU MAY NOT

O LORD, You have searched me and known me. You know when I sit down and when I rise up; You understand my thought from afar. You scrutinize my path and my lying down, and are intimately acquainted with all my ways. Even before there is a word on my tongue, Behold, O LORD, You know it all. - Psalm 139:1-4 (NIV)

For those who have dementia, there will be many times when other people do not understand the manifestations of the condition. It would be difficult to know what affected individuals feel, think and wish to communicate, or to fully appreciate what it is like to live with memory problems.

Often there may be times when people with dementia do not understand themselves or their own experiences. Difficulty communicating with others adds to the confusion they may experience.

Many family members and friends of those with dementia wish they knew what their loved ones were thinking or feeling, because they long to meet needs, make connections and provide help. But as dementia progresses and communication is more difficult, it becomes a challenge to continue to know the heart and mind of a loved one.

We should take comfort in the realization that there is One who knows and understands us completely, even more than we can understand ourselves. In fact, God understands us even when we cannot speak or do not seem to be capable of forming coherent thoughts. Read Psalm 139 and hear how God knows us now and across the span of time, from before birth and into the uncertainty of the future. There is nowhere we can be found which will escape the loving gaze of God. We are fully known by a loving God, even when we feel we don't know ourselves. Take courage and comfort in this truth: nothing can separate us from the love of God (Romans 8:38-39).

Lord, search me and know me when no one seems to understand me. Grant me the comfort of Your presence today, that I might find strength for today and hope for tomorrow. Amen.

Benjamin T. Mast, PhD (Reformed Christian/Baptist)

NO ACT OF LOVE IS EVER WASTED

But Jesus said, "Let her alone; why do you bother her? She has done a good deed to Me. "For you always have the poor with you, and whenever you wish you can do good to them; but you do not always have Me. "She has done what she could; she has anointed My body beforehand for the burial. "Truly I say to you, wherever the gospel is preached in the whole world, what this woman has done will also be spoken of in memory of her." - Mark 14:6-9 (NIV)

It had been a stressful, tense and volatile support group meeting. Several participants shared their sad stories of caring for loved ones with Alzheimer's. Some told how their loved ones had become distant and even belligerent. One person shook her head and said, "My husband just sits there with that blank look on his face and never says a mumbling word. I feel like I'm living alone." Another caregiver shared how her mother was living with a nephew who could not care for her. "I am at my wit's end," she said, "and I'm about to place Mom in a nursing home." Her comment made other members relive their guilt when they placed a loved one in a home. The tension was so thick you could cut it with a knife. As a facilitator, I used all my skills to turn the group around to a more positive feeling, but to no avail. For a moment we sat silently, depressed, not knowing what to say or do next.

Earlier I had given members of the group copies of our book, *No Act of Love is Ever Wasted*, but I doubt if any of the group had read much of the book. One member told me, "I am totally exhausted at the end of the day so I've had no time to read your book." Then, a flash of inspiration came to me, and I asked the group to listen to a poem, written by Jim Fowler, who himself was struggling with Alzheimer's. I opened my book to "They Will Remember," and slowly read these words:

> In those places of the heart, where soul still lurks, they will remember.
> In tactile hunger for hands that caress and care, they will remember.
> At heaven's gate where all the leaves of lost memories are restored,
> they WILL remember all the loving fragments, melodies, touches,
> prayers and tales by which you loved them.
> Angels will sing, dance and shout,
> sensing your love in those loved one's joys.

This poem redeemed that meeting. I felt that they realized their love was not wasted. They would be remembered.

God, show us that each inspired act of love performed helps to usher in Your Kingdom. Amen.

Richard L. Morgan, PhD, Retired Clergy (Presbyterian Church, USA)

BUSHELS OF PEAS

"Take my yoke upon you. Let me teach you, because I am humble and gentle at heart, and you will find rest for your souls. For my yoke is easy to bear, and the burden I give you is light." - Matthew 11:29-30 (NLT)

Which path shall I choose to walk today? Will today be a mental ferry ride into the past, visiting with friends long-since gone…or will today's journey reveal angry words and lost moments…frustration at the loss of independence for both my mom and me? The answer is soon revealed. Dementia has been kind today.

As I enter the nursing home room, my mom's sweet face shines back at me. "Guess what?" she eagerly shares. "I have been picking peas all day and Grandmama and I are exhausted!" I smile back at her and ask how many pints they canned and froze. She looks out the window and shares that she cannot remember but it was "a lot." While some would see this visit to the past as an opportunity to reorient to the present, I strive to see this as a blessing that Mama can find her way back home for a visit to the past.

As Mama's caregiver, her visit to the past is both a blessing and a reminder of things that will never be again. We will never together again sit on the porch, shelling peas and sharing stories. Mama taught me the fine art of canning vegetables and making sweet pear preserves. I wipe away the tears and recognize that it is a blessing that Mama can talk to those long-since gone and that those conversations are not to be corrected; rather, celebrated. It is now late August and the red-tinted ripe pears are falling from the old pear tree in my neighbor's yard…

Dear Lord, help me to remember that we are never alone on our journey, for You are with us always. Amen.

Laura Pannell, PhD, CPG (United Methodist)

REDEMPTIVE SUFFERING

"The pain that is brought into God's presence has a creative effect that enriches us for the rest of our lives. But the pain that is of man, borne in self-reliance and in a stoic fashion, repressing all emotion, brings death. In faith, we have the wonderful knowledge that we are never carrying the pain of caregiving on our own." - Dr. James Houston, Professor of Spiritual Theology, Regent College

I had the privilege of first hearing Dr. James Houston speak about ten years ago. A close friend of C. S. Lewis and one of the world's great theologians, Dr. Houston radiates a presence perceived in those who are enlivened by the Holy Spirit—his intellect is matched by humility and grace, freely shared with those who are fortunate enough to be found in his circle. My first encounter with him was enlightening, but subsequent interactions have been transformative.

Later I heard him speak at a conference on aging, this time about his experiences as caregiver for his wife, newly diagnosed with dementia. In this talk he put forth a theology of dementia, and spoke of intentional spirituality in the caregiving experience. Deeply moved by his ideas, afterward I made plans to travel to his Vancouver home for an on-camera interview to explore the persistence of personhood in those with dementia. The interview took place in April of 2012, portions of which will appear in a documentary produced by our foundation (Cognitive Dynamics) titled "Do You Know Me Now?"

"My dear," he said to his beloved wife, "these will be the best years of our lives." He spoke of the opportunity for spiritual growth emerging through physical affliction, that one's identity is both relational and God-given, and that one begins to become an elder as a child when the seeds of empathy are planted, later ripening in the caregiving experience. "I thank my wife and others with whom I am able to join in caretaking. They are bringing things out of me that are potentials for my own growth. Caregiving is a fruition of what we are meant to be." These are statements from a 90-year-old caregiver continuing to seek life-enrichment and spiritual growth in the day-to-day challenges, and calling, that is caregiving.

Dr. Houston is able to have this outlook because he has brought his sufferings "into God's presence," acknowledging that God has chosen to suffer alongside, even *inside* the lives we live. Pondering and living into such an earth-splitting reality is truly transformative, and enables us to be agents of transformation for those who are suffering with, and providing care for persons with dementia and Alzheimer's disease.

Suffering God, help to harken to the psalmist's words: "Cast thy burden upon the Lord, and He shall sustain thee." Amen. (Psalm 55:22 - KJV)

Daniel C. Potts, MD, FAAN, Elder (Presbyterian Church, USA)

LOVE COMES FULL CIRCLE

"Everything moves in circles. This is the way of life, and what we refuse to give we refuse to accept. Nothing is more important than we learn how to forgive both ourselves and others." - Ernest Holmes, Living in Science of Mind, 1984

There is something about his eyes. Yes, he is blind, and nearly 100 years old, but something behind his eyes still sparkles with life. At times, he is lucid. All at once he will begin the repetitive questions about finding his brother. I answer, "Dad, Wayne has been gone for the last twelve years." "Oh, I guess I knew that, but I thought he was up north in his car and that he would come by to see me."

"I'm going now, Dad, but I'll be back again very soon." We hug. He tells me how much he appreciates me, and we part. I know that before I get home there will be one or two phone messages asking me about his brother, or telling me he needs toothpaste, which I have just delivered.

I sigh and smile, because he is so sweet, and because I understand that this is the best I will have of him right now. This man who was my handsome, brilliant father, who was a driven and successful businessman, always striving for more, is now this humble, kind man who needs me so much.

I see this time of caregiving as a kind of forgiveness process. He wasn't a daddy I could talk to, but a stern father I had to measure up to. That was an impossible task, as he always demanded more than I could give.

Now he needs me, continuously tells me how much he loves me, and I simply love him back. It's a bit late for resentments or asking, "Where were you when I needed you?"

It is a gift to care for him. I am grateful that he lives in a residence where angels in human form tend to him with such graciousness. I know I am not equipped to do what they do every day. They have my deepest appreciation. Hands on or hands off, caring for a loved one who is slipping away a little more each day calls for reaching deeply within and accepting what is.

Love comes full circle. The father I yearned for years ago eluded me. The father I now care for has given me the gift of compassion and patience. When the last chapter of Dad's life is complete, I will be grateful for these years, and glad that I could be there to make them good for him.

Loving God, help me to let the old hurts and resentments fall away as I come full circle with my loved one. Through caregiving, grant that I may find the gift of loving-kindness, and help me to remain grateful. Amen.

Rev. Dr. Peggy Price, Center for Spiritual Living (Interdenominational)

WHEN IT FEELS LIKE GOD IS SILENT

He said, "Go out and stand on the mountain before the LORD, for the LORD is about to pass by." Now there was a great wind, so strong that it was splitting mountains and breaking rocks in pieces before the LORD, but the Lord was not in the wind; and after the wind an earthquake, but the LORD was not in the earthquake; and after the earthquake a fire, but the LORD was not in the fire; and after the fire a sound of sheer silence. - I Kings 19:11-15 (NIV)

One of the hardest times of struggle with Alzheimer's is after the confirming diagnosis becomes our reality measured in loss and decline. Though we resist thinking about it, inevitable questions creep in, like, "Where is God?" Grieving situations do this to us. Elijah was grieving and struggling with the same questions in this scripture text.

We start looking for small signs of normalcy. We become Elijah, knowing God will pass by, looking for an answer to our suffering in all the wrong places. We think surely God must be in the wind, looking for our beloved to recognize us. When we long for a good day with loved ones we are Elijah looking in the earthquake. We hope we can find solace by reading the news for the next cure; we are Elijah in the firestorm.

Elijah heard God only in the silence. How can God speak in the silence let alone be heard? In the silence we learn to hear a different voice. It is a voice of presence, felt rather than heard. In silence we realize it has been with us all along, though we have missed it. Just as Elijah only was able to hear God after everything else distracting him was silenced, because of the presence we begin to realize we aren't alone in our suffering. We begin to feel this presence as guidance and comfort.

Presence is what Elijah felt in the silence, in his aloneness. In the silence he heard God speaking because God's voice is not full of empty words like "there, there, everything will be ok." It is a voice beyond words, the voice of love which shares in suffering. In the silence God is suffering with us. The amazing thing is that this presence begins to be experienced in our loved one. It is the belief, the fleeting thought of God with us, which we only find because of the silence.

When we experience silence like Elijah's, we experience God not with our eyes and minds, but also with our essence and being, with our souls. It allows us to experience our loved one also in a new but different sense. Our sense of this presence comes in love and memory. Though in many ways our loved ones appear to be gone and God seems silent, our experience of God through our spirit has just begun.

O Divine One, when my grief distracts me and becomes too large for me to bear by myself, wrap Your strong arms around me so we can share the pain together, and its weight will not grow too heavy for me. Help me to feel Your presence in the silence and to hear Your voice. Amen.

Rev. Dr. William B. Randolph (United Methodist)

KIND FACES

As God's chosen ones, holy and beloved, clothe yourselves with compassion, kindness, humility, meekness, and patience. - Colossians 3:12

Often in my years as a social worker, caregivers have recounted their sadness when a loved one has dementia and does not know them or how they are related. This is especially difficult for those who are partners, children or good friends. We may give up trying to connect with a person with dementia who doesn't seem to recognize us. A wise woman taught me an alternative way to think about this. This valuable lesson has informed my relationships to this day, and provides a key precept for relating to those with dementia.

Maria lived in a long-term care facility. Dementia had taken its toll, and she would spend the day walking, seemingly aimlessly, around the facility. She said little, but smiled broadly when persons talked to her. She could not remember the names of her daily caregivers or her family. When her oldest son came nightly to visit her, they would take walks or go out for hamburgers. She seemed to delight in being with him.

During my work in that nursing home, I would frequently encounter Maria on her daily rounds. One night after her son had gone home, I gently inquired about the visit and who the man was that had been with her. She responded "I don't know, but I know that he was a kind man." This was at the time, and continues to be, a most important teaching; the kindness of another person connects even when recognition of the "facts" of that relationship fails.

Connecting "soul to soul" with another does not require full knowledge of that person's identity. What is essential is that we demonstrate kindness to each other. When persons are not able to recognize us as a particular person, they do know us by our kindness and love. Taking the time to remember a person as a precious child of God, and to truly share of ourselves is important. This requires great patience and gentleness. And we can try to understand the world in which a person with dementia lives. This requires lowliness and meekness.

We need kindness in our world and our relationships, and persons like Maria teach us its importance. Even if persons with dementia do not know our names or who we are, they know our kind faces when we take the time to be present to them.

Loving God, help us to put on kindness and patience as we serve those struggling with dementia. Assist us to become loving vessels of Your love. Open our hearts to learn from those who have much to teach. Amen.

Martha E. "Marty" Richards (Evangelical Lutheran Church in America)

COURAGE, HOPE, AND KINDNESS

"Courage is like love, it must have hope for nourishment." - Napoleon

I should not have been surprised; but, in fact, I was sideswiped when I learned my genetic status puts me at a 91% lifetime risk of getting Alzheimer's disease. For months, all I could think about was the caregiving responsibilities that my family had previously gone through with my great-grandmother, grandmother, two great uncles and my father who was in the middle stages of Alzheimer's. I was concerned about my family and also wondering who would LOVE me enough to embrace the responsibility of taking care of me. I feared for my future; and, like most caregivers who are overwhelmed with fears and frustrations, I withdrew into a deep dark hole trying to make sense of this disease and what possibly lay before me.

But, through counseling and prayer, I found courage and hope for a cure; and, in so doing, became more loving towards my father and kinder to myself, even with my genetic imperfection. Through this love, caregiving became easier and I was even able to find humor and patience in my father's new behaviors.

After my father became a resident at an assisted living facility, I would take him out on little outings. Forgetting that he had a propensity to take things that did not belong to him, I took him to the grocery store where he proceeded to fill a plastic bag with candy. I tried my best to stop him but to no avail. And that is when something beautiful happened. I approached the store manager and explained that my father had Alzheimer's disease, and that I would pay for whatever my father had confiscated. The manager gently smiled and said, "We know your father and we call that 'sampling!'" My father's illness gave the manager an opportunity to extend his kindness. And through his kindness I had hope that I also would be LOVED.

So, through this journey I realized that there is hope. There is so much more support than ever before for caregivers, and the kindness and understanding we extend to each other is invaluable. If we have the courage to come out of the shadows, we will be surprised at the love we receive in return. The knowledge of my genetic status became a blessing and my fear turned into courage and courage into hope. And, as I became more courageous through my hope, I was able to love my father and myself in a more patient and compassionate way.

Lord, please continue to be with me as You give me the strength and courage to carry on with my journey of hope to find a cure for Alzheimer's disease, the gift of compassion and understanding to help comfort caregivers, and the ability to bring inspiration to those who are affected by this disease. Thank you for Your blessing in gifting me with such a meaningful purpose. Amen.

Jamie Ten Napel Tyrone, RN (Interdenominational)

WINTER

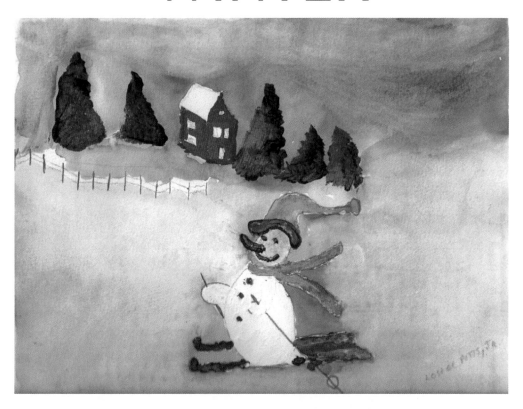

On the steel gray canvas of another winter with Alzheimer's disease, Lester's smiling snowman glides across baby blue powder with a pink scarf and a grin. Snowmen are not often encountered in Alabama winters, certainly not on skis, like this one. Maybe the frozen reality of Alzheimer's disease called out the inner boy for this make-believe escape to a happier time. Perhaps we can see that the snow brings an opportunity to put on our skis and keep moving along with the flow, though our faces may sting in the winter winds. We may not be certain where our loved ones have made their escape, but we must be prepared to go with them, clasping hands and warming spirits on the way. And as we join them in relationship, we may also find our own hearts "strangely warmed."

ON TRYING TO UNDERSTAND

Respect an elder who has lost his learning through no fault of his own. The fragments of the Tablets broken by Moses were kept in the Ark of the Covenant alongside the new.
- Babylonian Talmud; Berachot 8b

I am surrounded by mystery. I am encased in a puzzle. How has this happened? Why has this occurred? This person, once so filled with life, before me now as someone broken? Our tradition tells us that the broken fragments of the first set of tablets that Moses brought to the people were preserved in the ark with the new tablets. As I sit here thinking of what was, I cannot help but wonder what is being preserved.

In a silent scream I call out, trying to understand the reason for this. How to make sense of this reality, how to honor and respect the soul that I love. Is this a hint, perhaps? In the midst of this mystery, this puzzle, we are left with the gift of love. Perhaps we can come to understand that even in this sadness, the possibility of love is never out of reach and that, in the end, it is love that is our greatest gift, the missing piece of life's puzzle.

How can this all make sense? It may be revealed in the passage of time as mysteries are often revealed; slowly, and with a faith that meaning will ultimately be secured. In that spirit, read this poem by Rabbi Lawrence Kushner, which can remind us that each of us contains within us a spark of divinity, and that each of us contains a piece of an eternal puzzle that celebrates the mystery of our relationships and the power of our love.

> **Each lifetime is the pieces of a jigsaw puzzle**
> For some there are more pieces. For others the puzzle is more difficult to assemble.
> Some seem to be born with a nearly completed puzzle. And so it goes.
> Souls trying this way and that; trying to assemble the myriad parts.
> But know this. No one has within themselves all the pieces to his or her puzzle.
> Like before the days they used to seal jigsaw puzzles in cellophane,
> Insuring that all the pieces were there, everyone carries within them at least one and probably many pieces to someone else's puzzle. Sometimes they know it.
> Sometimes they don't. And when you present your piece
> which is worthless to you, to another, whether you know it or not,
> Whether they know it or not, you are a messenger from the Most High.

Heal us Eternal and we shall be healed, save us and we shall be saved. Grant full healing to our wounds, our illness, our pain. Blessed are YOU, Eternal, Healer of the sick. (Traditional prayer from the daily prayer book on healing; a spiritual healing, as the prayer does not mention a "cure.")

Rabbi Richard F. Address (Jewish)

"I COME TO THE END... I AM STILL WITH YOU"

If I rise on the wings of the dawn, if I settle on the far side of the sea, even there your hand will guide me, your right hand will hold me fast. If I say, "Surely the darkness will hide me and the light become night around me," even the darkness will not be dark to you; the night will shine like the day, for darkness is as light to you. - Psalm 139:9-12 (NIV)

Meryl and Hugh introduced me to Alzheimer's forty years ago. Back then the illness was not well known. But Hugh, a devoted husband instinctively made decisions about Meryl's care. She had been an elegant and proud woman. Hugh brought her to church as long as he could, but eventually she became very dependent on him. Their morning routine took longer and longer. The day came when he could not get her fed, bathed, and dressed in time for church. Hugh hired some help. But he still wanted to be with her all he could.

Recently married, I observed the greatest love story I'd ever known. I was being tutored in the meaning of love. Serving my first parish, I was taught many things by this 70-year-old caregiver and his beautiful wife who never remembered me. Though I was barely 27, Hugh allowed me to be their pastor. He talked to me about his journey and the stresses of life; about his grief, devotion, love and determination to keep Meryl at home.

It was a Sunday night, the week before Christmas. Our little parish of three churches had scheduled to go caroling. It turned so bitterly cold that good sense would have said, "Cancel." But a handful of the faithful showed up. We decided to go and sing for Meryl and Hugh, who had not been to church since spring. Hugh insisted we come in out of the cold. We visited briefly. Meryl was behaving like a flirtatious 13 year old, and kept asking if we knew her boyfriend (Hugh), exhibiting other childlike behaviors. Hugh settled her on the sofa beside him and told her we were going to sing for them.

"Silent Night, Holy Night," we sang. I will never forget the tears that began to slip down Meryl's cheeks, the look of recognition on her face, the deep connection we all felt in that holy moment, the level ground on which we stood. There we were, a motley crew, each broken and gazing into the manger at the "light that overcomes the darkness."

Holy God, thank you for allowing our feet of clay to rest upon ground made holy by Your gracious presence. From where we stand, we cannot see the dark places where Your light penetrates and memory never fades; where Your love never fails nor pauses. We are thankful for glimpses of Your power at work, bringing light into darkness, hope into despair, strength to the weak, and life out of death. Holy God, lead me by Your hand today to Holy Ground. Amen.

Reverend Brenda F. Carroll (United Methodist)

WHEN FRUSTRATION IS GETTING THE BETTER OF YOU

Be still, and know that I am God - Psalm 46:10

Bill and Paul have been together for decades and were recently married. Bill loves going on fishing trips. The last time Paul told Bill that they were going on a fishing trip, Bill was excited and went into the garage and asked, "Shouldn't we pack the cooler for the trip?" Paul answered, "Yes, but the trip is next weekend. We can wait a few days."

Some minutes later, Bill asked from the garage, "Shouldn't we pack the cooler?" And Paul said, "The trip is next weekend. It's only Monday today." This answer satisfied Bill for a few minutes, after which he asked, still in the garage, "Shouldn't we pack the cooler?"

If you recognize yourself and your loved one in this exchange, if you know what it's like to want to laugh and scream and cry and pull out your hair all at the same time, then know you're not alone. After you answer the same question for the fourth or fifth time, catch yourself before you answer again, and take a deep breath. Then a second deep breath. And then a third. Remember God saying, "Be still, and know that I am God."

Paul says that he has a three-answer limit now, after which he tries to distract Bill with something else. When Paul gets irritated, he gives that irritated part of him a time out and tells himself, "The disease is asking the same question incessantly, not Bill."

Dear Healer of All Healers, Be with Bill and Paul and those like them who need Your calm, Your peace, and Your serenity right now. Be with them in the easier times and in the harder times. Let them lean on You and on Your strength when no other human is around. And let us say, "Amen."

Rabbi Susan S. Conforti (Jewish)

HOW TO AVOID EVER-NEW GRIEF

Thou Shalt Not Deal Falsely with One Another - Deuteronomy 19:11 (Tanakh)

Not knowing any better, when we started out and Dave was in the hospital, we told Sally the truth, or at least the truth as we wished it to be. When Sally asked, "Where is Dave?" we'd answer, "Dave is sick, but he's coming home soon." When Dave died, we stayed with untarnished truth. When Sally asked, "Where is Dave?" we answered, "Dave has died." During the service for Dave and during the graveside burial service, Sally kept crying.

I have officiated at many memorials, funerals, and burials, and it's always difficult when one of the principal mourners has Alzheimer's or another brain disease that causes dementia. Sally was one of those mourners. Her husband of over fifty years had just died, and Sally was understandably sad.

I consoled myself by thinking that once Sally sees Dave's casket go down into the grave, then Sally will have to understand that Dave has died. As you could have guessed, Sally's remembrance of Dave's funeral ended the moment we returned to our cars. Not two blocks away from the cemetery, we heard the question, "Where is Dave?" yet again.

Letting Sally know that Dave is dead was only causing Sally to hear the news again as if for the first time—her pain and shock and grief was fresh and new each every time we told her. Someone finally realized that our truthful answer was unnecessarily painful. Now when Sally asks, "Where is Dave?" we all know how to answer. We say, "He's not here right now, but you'll see him soon." Our revised response is just as truthful, and it avoids breaking the news to Sally that—yet again for us, but ever-new for Sally—Dave is dead. I'm all for being truthful and also for eschewing inflicting unnecessary pain, and I'm thrilled we don't have to put Sally through any more heartache.

Dear Healer of All Healers, be with us as we learn to communicate with our beloved brothers and sisters who are always in an eternal present. May we value them even more highly for their abilities to be here now. And let us all say, "Amen."

Rabbi Susan S. Conforti (Jewish)

"HERE I AM LORD..."

Then I heard the voice of the Lord saying, "Whom shall I send? And who will go for us?" And I said, "Here am I. Send me!" - Isaiah 6:8

When serving the critically ill in a ministerial role, the question of praying for a miracle often presents itself. If we believe in the power of prayer and the presence of miracles, then isn't a primary charge of the caregiver to never take away hope?

I was a little surprised recently when visiting a patient for the first time who had been living for a while with a terminal diagnosis. She had been coping with her illness for several years, and appeared to have experienced the kind of grieving that Dr. Elisabeth Kübler-Ross described in her landmark book, *On Death and Dying*. There was more resignation in our conversation than I expected. When the subject of prayer came up, and I was ready to focus on a prayer for healing, she declared, "I don't pray for miracles any more—though I would take one if God had it coming to me. Now I pray that I can be a messenger."

This person prided herself in being able to model her faith to those who looked upon her mostly with sadness, fear and trepidation. She hoped that her faith and courage, and even her resignation, could "be a beacon" to those around her. She wanted people to know that her faith was helping her to persevere through the pain and fear, and to peaceful acceptance of her coming death.

Another person who seemed to arrive at this point was Pope John Paul II, who struggled mightily with his Parkinson's disease for a long time. It seemed clear to those around him near the end that he wanted people to know the role his faith was playing in his demeanor and perseverance. He wanted to be a messenger in his last days, a "beacon of light" on the sanctity of life and the power of faith, even in the face of pain. He knew prayers for miracles were important, but wanted to model the role of a faithful servant to the end.

Is God calling some of us to take on this heavy mantle and witness through an illness to the power of faith? Will our response be, "Here I am, Lord. Send me?"

This may not be an easy place for caregivers and family members to go…they may not have arrived at that peaceful resignation. But this attitude can be a huge gift to those who survive the passing of a loved one.

Heavenly Father, give us caregivers the grace to be able to go where our loved one is. Help us to respect their resignation and witness even when we are still struggling with the gravity of their condition. If theirs is a role of messenger and beacon, help us to walk on the path which they are illuminating, and to help others walk that path as well. "Here I am, Lord. Send me!" Amen.

Deacon Michael Francis Curren (Roman Catholic)

STRONGER WHERE WE HAVE BEEN WEAK

But he said to me, "My grace is sufficient for you, for power is made perfect in weakness." So, I will boast all the more gladly of my weaknesses, so that the power of Christ may dwell in me. Therefore I am content with weaknesses, insults, hardships, persecutions, and calamities for the sake of Christ; for whenever I am weak, then I am strong. - 2 Corinthians 12:9-10

When I have been called to be with families who are living through issues of dementia with their parents, there can be an overriding sense of never-ending brokenness. With some illnesses, there is hope, and with others there is inevitable progression to death. But with dementia, we live with brokenness for so long it seems like it can be never-ending. And then there is the guilt that we can all feel when we wish the brokenness could just be over.

In my spare time I work as a hobbyist, building things or repairing things made of wood. One day, after gluing and clamping two pieces together, I read the words printed on the bottle of glue. What I saw there made me smile. It said that if the glue is used properly, and the broken piece or new joint is clamped properly and allowed the appropriate time to set, then the wood will actually become stronger where it had been joined, splintered or weakened. Imagine that.

I have witnessed that this is indeed possible, even probable, for those who can turn to their faith at times of despair. Like my wood pieces, it does not happen quickly—it takes patience and faith. It takes more time than we would like to give it.

We don't know the weakness with which the Apostle Paul lived. It really doesn't matter. In Christ, Paul found his weakness turn to strength. He found strength, through faith, in that weakness. In a strange way, that weakness became a blessing. It became a source of perseverance, and as Paul tells us in Romans 5, perseverance brings hope and hope does not disappoint, for in it God, through the Holy Spirit, has poured himself out into our hearts!

Heavenly Father, when we have our moments of despair and brokenness, give us the grace to remember to turn to You—to see the blessing that Your love for us truly is, and give us the renewed strength to be healed even where we are weak and broken. Amen.

Deacon Michael Francis Curren (Roman Catholic)

WHEREVER WE ARE

"Oh LORD, You have searched me and You know me; even the darkness will not be dark to You." - Psalm 139:1, 12 (NIV)

As I watched her walk in the door I could read by her body language that she was struggling. Katherine's husband has dementia, attending the respite ministry I direct for the past year.

Fred has a unique medical history—muscular dystrophy (MD) coupled with dementia. Theirs is a fairly new marriage of seven years. She knew about the MD but the dementia began after their marriage. Their love is precious yet so tested in this young union. Katherine deals with depression, so when the stress of caregiving gets too much, she begins a downward spiral where she just wants to sleep and shut away the pain. This day her stress is palpable; from her disheveled appearance and slump of her shoulders to the pain in her eyes.

The ministry of Grace Arbor is three-fold ministering to the person with dementia by care, the caregiver by respite, and the older adult volunteers by service.

Smiles and hugs are shared with Katherine from my volunteers. Fred is whisked away to the table by another volunteer carefully assisting him as he walks jerkily on his walker. Katherine watches with tear-filled eyes.

Laying a comforting hand on her shoulder, I invite her into the other room for a brief heart checkup—listening and then prayer. The tears fall freely and I allow her to unload the burden she has been hauling around that morning like a stone on her chest. I then grab her hand and ask if I can pray for her. The best gift I can give a caregiver is the assurance they are not alone and the reminder of Jesus' presence with them.

Spirit words are spoken and off she goes out the door—shoulders a little higher, empowered by Jesus' love. I breathe a thankful prayer to the One who is always present—the Psalmist reminds us that even the darkness is not dark when exposed to the light of God's love.

Father God, You love Your children, promising never to leave or forsake them. I ask that You would remind these precious caregivers of these truths. Meet them at their place of need so that they will be filled with peace, strength, comfort and joy. Thank You for Your love, in Jesus' holy name, Amen.

Robin Dill, Director, Grace Arbor (United Methodist)

"THIS TOO SHALL PASS"

Those who are insulted but do not insult, hear themselves reviled but do not answer... of them the Scriptures say, "May God's friends be as the sun going forth in its might." - Judges 5:31 (Talmud, Tractate Shabbat 88b)

These words comforted Ma for 84 of her 87 years. Whenever she faced a challenge—a recalcitrant child, an overcooked dinner, a flat tire on an isolated road, an illness of a loved one—she repeated, "This too shall pass"—and it did. Although Ma could not prevent bad things from happening to me, she could assure me that I would survive.

And then Ma got dementia, and I lost my faith in her lifelong slogan. Instead of passing like an unwelcome storm, Ma's confusion worsened until she became dangerous to herself. Dad and I had no choice but to place her in a facility.

We visited daily. Though the home had its own staff, I discovered that people with dementia are often overlooked. Aides sometimes lack the patience to handle questions repeated in the same monotone or with belligerence that can develop in one whose mind has become like an unfocused picture. Therefore, I became Ma's aide—doing for her things which my healthy mother would never have permitted: cleaning and diapering her; seeing her without dentures when I had to clean her teeth; feeding her—the woman who never snacked—cookies and chips she craved.

Some days Ma would smile when she saw me and hold my hand; on others she would call me a "piece of shit," curl into the fetal position, and refuse to look at me or speak. This was not the mother who nourished us delectably at Thanksgiving with Toll House cookies and delicate-as-air lemon pies. This was not the woman who tended to her customers at the children's store with expertise, experience and enthusiasm. While the rest of us slept, she ate breakfast, did laundry and dusted. Before others arrived at the store, she had prepared coffee, gone through layaways and organized everything for the day.

Ma seemed too feisty for dementia; too smart—she could mentally add her grocery bill and remember every detail from books she read. Dementia stole the last three years of Ma's life, turning me from daughter to caregiver, my love replaced by resentment, frustration and fear. Dementia did not end until it claimed Ma's life.

Then it began again with Dad. I now care for my 98-year-old father who remembers hazily and converses illogically. Thanks to experience, I deal with Dad patiently and with understanding. I do not welcome dementia, but have learned to accept it.

Lord, we don't know why bad things happen; only that You're not the cause. Constant Companion, please take away bad memories, replacing them with reminders of a life well lived. Give grace to mourn losses and live in hope. Amen.

Ronna L. Edelstein (Jewish)

REMEMBER MY PAST

Therefore, as God's chosen people, holy and dearly loved, clothe yourselves with compassion, kindness, humility, gentleness and patience. - Colossians 3:12 (NIV)

It is common for us to believe that it is the caregiver who suffers the most. I don't know that I agree. With dementia, everyone suffers. All you need do is take a "Virtual Dementia Tour" to glimpse how difficult it must be for the person with the diagnosis.

There's a poignant document circulating on Facebook, called "Ten Requests from a Dementia Journeyer." It encourages us to look beyond the illness and treat the individual with patience and loving kindness. Of the ten requests, one that especially resonates with me is, "Remember my past - for I was once a healthy, vibrant person full of life, love and laughter with abilities and intelligence."

When I moved my husband Richard to assisted living I prepared his biography to be included in his chart. I wanted his attendants to know that he was so much more than who they saw before them. I wanted them to have a glimpse of the great man that he was—his considerable accomplishments, his many interests, his sense of humor, his generosity...

Richard was hospitalized in November 2011 as a result of medication side effects and dehydration. He was taken to the hospital late at night and when we arrived, two friends, both pastors, were in the emergency room to greet us and to offer support and assistance through the administrative maze. Obviously they recognized the value of human life, even in the most compromised of situations, and were unconcerned that their visit would most certainly, on a cognitive level, be forgotten.

During this hospitalization my husband's condition deteriorated, and he plummeted from mid-stage to late-stage dementia. Richard died exactly four months to the day he was admitted to the hospital. In between, there were five hospital transfers. That's a story for another time; one that sadly underscores the lack of late-stage care available to many.

During that hospital stay, we were visited by the chaplain. She asked about Richard's life, his contributions and accomplishments. Later we prayed together, not just for strength for what lay before us, but in thanksgiving for the man he had been. I will never forget that kindness.

Heavenly Father, please allow us to look beyond the mask of dementia to see and appreciate the person who remains. Let us not forget this person's contributions, for this very simple kindness validates not just the individual with dementia, but all who love and cherish him. Amen.

Lynda Everman (United Methodist)

BETRAYAL

I have told you these things, so that in me you may have peace. In this world you will have trouble. But take heart! I have overcome the world. - John 16.33 (NIV)

I couldn't explain to my mother where Dad had gone. For several weeks he'd had confusing symptoms of weakness, twice falling in his living room, once cutting his head. He was 97 and of sound mind, so this sudden change in his demeanor was frightening.

But once he was hospitalized, it was determined he needed rehabilitation for several weeks. So he was moved to a nursing home and I began to drive my mother from home to see him. At this point in their lives they were still quite independent. I saw them once a week, or less, but had begun to notice their being in greater need of support which, predictably, they didn't want to accept.

When Dad was in rehabilitation, I stayed with my Mom two nights, commuting on to my work 30 miles away, and then returning in the late afternoon to fix her dinner and see that she got herself safely to bed. The third night I brought her to our house for a change of scenery (so I could stay in my own bed!). But it was clear she became more confused every day she spent out of the routine in her own home.

In the morning she took her pills handily from her plastic pill caddy and we drove 20 minutes north, stopping by their home to pick up more of her things. I opened the back door, and she stepped in, asking, "Carl? Dad? Are you home?" She broke my heart. She couldn't remember where he was.

I explained to her again as we drove to the home for our visit. When Mom went in to talk with Dad, I asked the nurse for help in discerning whether Mother could support herself. She clearly wasn't managing on her own. When they agreed, I moved my mom—without her permission—out of her home into the same facility with my dad.

"Cathy, I don't want to stay here," she began, angrily, as she sat staring at me in the admissions office in a red blouse, black cardigan and slacks.

"I know, Mom, but it won't be for long. When Dad is stronger you can both be moved to an apartment," I said as if I knew, yet wondering if that would even be possible.

"I want to go home," she answered defiantly. Ironically, acting in what I felt was her best interest, I made sure she couldn't. Unfortunately, such heart-rending decisions are common in the lives of caregivers. So we cling to our faith for answers and strength.

God of Strength and Comfort, help me trust that in the times I cannot know what is best, I will find You here beside me, giving me strength. Amen.

The Rev. Catherine Fransson (American Baptist)

REJECTION

I remain confident of this: I will see the goodness of the Lord in the land of the living. Wait for the Lord; be strong and take heart and wait for the Lord.- Psalm 27:13-14 (NIV)

After being advised to give my mother some time to adjust to her new surroundings in this nursing home, I stay away several days, hoping she is making peace with her new room, the pictures I've hung, the stuffed rabbit, and places on her dresser for her jewelry, what little I've been told is wise to leave.

I drive in and park the car, letting myself into the main lobby where I look for her as well as in the day room, to no avail. So I head for her room down the hall.

There she greets me with a lined face full of worry. "I need to go home, Cathy. Dad may need me now, and I don't know where he is."

The walls were bare. She had taken everything down I had hung up, and rolled up the framed pictures of her and Dad, her grandkids and a lovely sketch of a cat she was fond of, in her pajamas and underwear, and stuffed them into the drawers of her dresser.

"But Mom, Dad is here; we'll go see him in a minute. Don't you want these pictures up so you feel at home?"

"It's long since time we headed home. Tell your dad we need to get off this ship and open up the house. We've been away too long."

I couldn't dissuade her from the image she had in her mind of being on a cruise ship far too long. She couldn't wait to get home.

I did convince her to come with me into the hall in the other direction and find Dad in his own room by himself. We sat down for a while, but he was having none of it. Her confusion frightened and embarrassed him. His response was to look the other way.

When I left, I thought, I have not made either one of them more comfortable than they were. What good is it for me to come? But then, how can I stay away? I had no good answer. And I was miserable.

God, my Light and Salvation, help me to trust that even when I do not know what will help, my presence, with Your Spirit, is enough. Amen.

The Rev. Catherine Fransson (American Baptist)

CONFRONTING OUR MORTALITY

There is a time for everything, and a season for every activity under heaven: a time to be born and a time to die... - Ecclesiastes 3:1-2 (NIV)

I am middle aged and, like many in my situation, I have my share of health issues. But I am always puzzled when someone whom I consider to be a person of deep faith tells me, "My aches and pains are alright, considering the alternative." As a Christian who takes his beliefs seriously, I, frankly, consider the alternative to be rather nice.

We live in a death-denying society, a society in which the young and attractive are the ideal and the elderly are often marginalized. Families will often refuse to acknowledge that their loved one is dying and insist that all possible measures be taken to keep her alive, even if she appears to have no quality of life. To many, including many physicians, death can represent failure and treatment is continued long after any rational hope of cure has vanished and the treatment only prolongs intense suffering.

Facing Alzheimer's forces us to confront our own mortality. This can be a very good thing. It may allow us room to think about what kind of death we want, what measures we will allow to keep ourselves alive when our condition is terminal. It may help us be more loving in the present knowing that one day we will have to say goodbye to those we hold dear. It may help us make adequate provision for our own old age, and, yes, our own possible dementia.

Few like to think about end of life issues, but being a caregiver for someone with Alzheimer's makes it prudent to start planning for this eventuality. And planning for the end of life should be an important matter for us all.

Lord, may we never hide from our mortality, but recognizing that death is as much a part of life as birth, we may provide wisely for the future; and, when the time comes that we shall die, we may face death with that peace that comes only from You in whose embrace we shall rest securely forever. Amen.

The Rev. Dr. Michael Gemignani (Episcopal)

GOD IN THE DARKNESS

The Lord is close to the broken hearted and saves those who are crushed in spirit.
- Psalm 34:18 (NIV)

He has sent me to bind up the broken hearted, to proclaim freedom for the captives
and release from darkness for the prisoners - Isaiah 61:1 (NIV)

Was my beloved wife Nilda, who was living in the shadows of Alzheimer's, closer to God than I, her caretaker? There were times when I wondered. I was the one who was brokenhearted and crushed in spirit as I was losing the wonderful woman whom I had taken for better or worse, in sickness and in health. The commitment and love our vows embodied was being etched on my soul every day as Nilda slid ever more closely toward death. She was the captive of a terrible darkness from which the only release is death. And, yet, I sensed—no, I knew— that God was present, not just to me living in the "real" world, nor just to her living in a world of illusion, but to both of us in a magnificent, almost palpable, way; a way that proclaimed freedom and release in a situation that could have, would have, destroyed us were it not for that holy presence.

Yes, sometimes it is hard to see God standing close by because we are blinded by tears. And it may be hard to see God dwelling within someone we love who can no longer respond to our questions, who may not even recognize who we are. And that is why is it so important not to pray, "Lord, why has this happened to us?" but to pray, "Lord, let us see Your presence in this darkness."

Life, I believe, is a school to teach us to love. It is more difficult to love in times of adversity than in times of happiness, but the lessons that can be learned in suffering are more profound and more lasting. These are lessons that God can use to bring us to holiness.

God, You are indeed close to the brokenhearted and You save those who are crushed in spirit. Now, in this time of suffering, both for myself as caregiver and for the loved one for whom I care, give us a sense of Your presence, for we know You are with us in our pain. Give my loved one peace in her affliction and teach us each to love as You would have us love that we might be all that You would have us be. Amen.

The Rev. Dr. Michael Gemignani (Episcopal)

WHEN ALL SEEMS LOST

She had suffered under the care of many doctors and had spent all she had, yet instead of getting better she grew worse. - Mark 5:25-26 (NIV)

Elie Wiesel tells the story of a group of Jewish people imprisoned in a concentration camp during World War II who decided to put God on trial for failing to live up to His promises to protect them. There was a lot of evidence presented by the lawyers—one for God, one for the people. After all the presentations and deliberations, the verdict was read and God was found guilty.

"Now what do we do?" they wondered, after sitting in silence.

The only answer that made sense was to pray.

This story was read and discussed at a retreat for church women that I lead. They didn't understand why these people would turn to prayer after the verdict.

Shortly after this retreat, I was leading worship in the continuing care facility where I work and I shared with that group of faithful people the story Elie Wiesel had told. They understood it immediately, knowing that prayer is the only appropriate response when you have lost everything, including what you have believed about God.

We sat in this truth, joining ourselves with others who have turned to God in the face of devastating loss. This community understands that faith begins when you have nothing.

Gracious God, embrace us when we have nothing, when all else has failed. We desire to be Your people, relinquishing all in order to be found in You. Amen.

Rev. Barbara J. "Bobbie" Hineline (The United Church of Christ)

THE GREATEST TEACHER

"If you go more deeply into your own spiritual practice, you will encounter the suffering of others again and again, and you will have the capacity to acknowledge it, respond to it, and feel deep compassion." - His Holiness the Dalai Lama, The Path to Tranquility, 1999

How could I ever have guessed that some of the most heartening experiences arose amidst the most difficult situations? My husband Harrison, known as Hob, was suffering from the losses of dementia when he began having mini-stokes, often in public places. He'd pass out, someone would call 911, and each time I'd be sure he was dying.

We were fortunate. The combination of Hob's teaching the course on Death and Dying at our local university and his many years of meditation practice led to his being exceptionally open to the subject of death—even his own.

One time, as he lay in the back of the ambulance, the EMTs were yelling at him, trying to break through his unconsciousness. "Harrison, can you hear us? Can you hear us?"

I saw him stir and then he replied, "Will you guys please keep it down? I'm trying to die here."

What a startling statement! Surely the first time EMTs had heard such a request. Yet given the depth of his spiritual practice, his words didn't surprise me; they arose from his deep acceptance of death.

The next day, he began reflecting on his near death experience.

"I was going to all these places I haven't previously visited. And now that I've died once, I can use that as my guide. This passing out, it's simple. There's nothing scary here. In fact, it's just fine. If dying is this easy—no problem."

Whether the subject of death comes up with our loved one, or not, with dementia or any illness, we're constantly asked to let go and have faith. An enormous challenge. As I used to say to Hob, "We need to trust that we can do this together"—an affirmation of his dignity, no matter how impaired he might become—and a statement about faith. In his last year when his memory for poetry was still intact, he quoted,

"Life and death on one tether, and running beautifully together."

May we have the faith and strength to meet whatever arises and trust that love is stronger than death. Amen.

Olivia Ames Hoblitzelle (Buddhist)

I AM HERE FOR YOU!

And serve God and ascribe nothing as partner unto Him. (Show) kindness and compassion unto parents, unto near kindred, orphans, the needy, unto the neighbor who is of kin (to you) and the neighbor who is not of kin, the fellow-traveler, the wayfarer and those whom you are responsible by oaths. God loves not who is arrogant and boastful! - The Noble Quran, 4:36

When I moved to California I was pregnant with my first child and in dire need of support and care due to my difficult pregnancy. My brother-in-law's parents treated me as their own daughter and provided me with everything I needed. They became my family and I became their daughter, and with the passing of time, my three kids called them "Grandpa" and "Grandma."

A few years ago, the father was diagnosed with Alzheimer's. This wasn't easy to deal with, since he was known as the grandfather of the whole community, and his home was always warmly open—hosting dinners and brunches for over twenty-five families during holidays and Holy Days. Most of the time, children could be found happily running down the stairs; boys playing games in the garage and girls hiding in the bedroom, talking and sharing secrets. Men gathered in the backyard grilling assorted meats, and women in the kitchen prepared the rest of the meal. It felt like home, sharing these days with everyone. We were all one big family.

Grandpa was starting to forget things, as well as people, and he was getting frustrated with that. Over time, as his situation worsened, visits were limited to family and close friends. He received the best care and love that any father can get from his two sons and daughter, who moved across the street from her parents' home to be closer to him and offer care. Whenever I visited him, they would spend time reminding him who I am—Maria, married to the doctor, from the old stories.

As time passed, Grandpa became more and more fatigued. He spent most of his time in his room sleeping, despite whoever came to visit him. Interestingly, his daughter said that the only time Grandpa ever left his room was when he was told that my father was outside waiting for him. Grandpa wasn't only my brother-in-law's uncle, but he was also my daddy's good friend!

Her words brought tears to my eyes and made me realize what love Grandpa carried for my dad. Even more, it made me recognize how valued and significant my presence was for Grandpa and his whole family. People who struggle with dementia may not remember the present, but they have strong memories and beauties of the past that they will hold on to until the last minute of their lives, like Grandpa did.

Dear Lord! I am grateful for the health You granted me, the family and friends You gave me. I humble myself and ask You to protect and be with them when they are in need, as they were there for me. I humble myself and pray that You make me a tool of joy in the life of those whom You choose for me to serve, and I humble myself and ask You to help me recognize the favors that people bestowed on me, regardless of how big or how small. Amen.

Maria Khani, Educator and Spiritual Counselor (Muslim)

THE NATIVITY PLAY

You shall love the Lord your God with all your heart, with all your soul, and with all your might. - Deuteronomy 6:5 (Tanakh)

Noticing a sudden, significant decline in Dorothy's cognitive abilities, her children decided to insure the upcoming Christmas holiday would be as uplifting as possible. A year earlier, dementia had made it necessary for Dorothy—the matriarch of a large family—to move to a senior residential care center.

An amiable, genteel woman, she flourished in her new home—participating in activities and regularly attending the weekly worship service where she relished singing old hymns and reciting the Lord's Prayer and Psalm 23. She was friendly with staff and her fellow residents, her social skills compensating for cognitive losses she had sustained.

But recently, both family members and staff had begun to notice Dorothy's worsening confusion and that she needed more cuing regarding "activities of daily living." Wondering if this was a sign that her days on earth might be numbered, Dorothy's family decided that if this Christmas was going to be her last one, it would be an inspiring experience for her—and a memorable one for them.

The festivities began with Dorothy and her family attending the Christmas Eve program at the church where Dorothy had been a longtime, faithful member. Wanting her to focus solely on the program without distractions from the sights and around her, they made sure to sit on the first row.

When the program—a re-enactment of the Nativity—began, the transformation in Dorothy was immediate. To their great joy, her family saw how the play mesmerized her—eyes sparkling, face aglow in anticipation, as she connected with countless memories of similar scenes over the years. Then it happened:

One of the shepherds approached the manger and exclaimed, "Is this baby the one we have waited for? Is this infant the Promised One? Is he really the true Messiah?"

In the blink of an eye—and to the astonishment of all around her—Dorothy leaped out of her seat and, in a mixture of passionate affirmation and annoyance, shouted back:

"OF COURSE HE IS! ANY DUMB SON OF A BITCH KNOWS THAT!!"

Heavenly Father, In Your wisdom and mercy, You have given us mental, emotional and spiritual abilities with which we may know and love You. With passing years, if these abilities fade, we echo the Psalmist: "Cast me not off when I am old; when my strength fails, do not forsake me." Grant our spirits strength, that we may continue to hear Your voice and feel Your touch. Amen.

Rabbi Cary Kozberg (Jewish)

EMBRACING GRIEF: THERE IS NO GREATER SORROW

"There is no greater sorrow than to remember happiness in a time of misery." -
Dante, The Inferno

One day when I was visiting Ed, my beloved Romanian life partner of 30 years, in the memory care facility where he lived, they were having a festive sing-along. I sat down beside him to keep him company.

All of a sudden the activity director, singing at the top of her lungs and pounding away on the piano, ripped into a rendition of the Beatles' song, *Yesterday*. I was caught off guard, completely unprepared for the torrent of emotions it would bring about.

Yes, yesterday all my troubles *had* seemed so far away. And yes, now they *were* here to stay. Ed wasn't ever going to get better. Tears welled up in my eyes and I bit my lip as I tried to keep from bursting into tears.

Then more words tumbled out and intensified my sorrow. In some ways Ed *wasn't* half the man he used to be. There *was* a shadow hanging over him. The pain was searing.

Memories of yesterdays shared long ago suddenly flashed before my eyes. I remembered our first date. How we'd met and fallen in love that beautiful summer. I remembered the pet names we called each other. Cuddling on the sofa and talking into the wee hours of the morning. I remembered Ed's ever gallant and chivalrous manners. How he used to sneak into my house on my birthday while I was at work and leave flowers on my dining room table. I remembered our exciting trips to Hilton Head and Italy.

Suddenly I realized I could no longer control myself. I knew that in a matter of seconds I'd be crying like a baby so I jumped up and left because I didn't want to make a scene in front of the staff and the other residents.

I drove home on autopilot, crying uncontrollably all the way. But it was a good cry. It was the first time I'd cried about Ed's condition. The first time I'd cried about my loss of my constant supporter. My biggest fan. My chief confidant. And the first time I realized how very much I had loved him and still loved him.

By the time I arrived home I was better. I had gotten in touch with my grief, acknowledged it, and given myself permission to feel it deeply. And that felt good.

Dear Lord, help me accept and embrace my sorrow that I may find comfort in my time of grief. Amen.

Marie Marley, PhD (Interdenominational)

SHARING GIFTS OF FRIENDSHIP

I do not call you servants any longer, because the servant does not know what the master is doing; but I have called you friends, because I have made known to you everything that I have heard from my Father. - John 15:15

Dementia is sometimes termed "a disease of exclusion" because cherished friends so often fall away, muttering excuses ("He's not really here anymore," "I want to remember her as she was").

Because we over-privilege cognition as defining selfhood ("I think, therefore I am"), we conclude that we cannot continue our friendship if our friend is no longer fully a "self." But Jesus, who named us His friends, calls us to maintain our friendships with one another no matter what our circumstances or conditions. Indeed, it is through our relationships, not our cognitive ability, that our very identity as a person is formed and maintained.

Meister Eckhart, in describing the Trinity, wrote "When the Father laughs to the Son and the Son laughs back to the Father, that laughter gives pleasure, that pleasure gives joy, that joy gives love, and that love gives the persons of the Trinity, of whom the Holy Spirit is one." God's very being is defined by relationship, and we are created to be in relationship with God and with one another. In these relationships we are to share the gifts of laughter, pleasure, joy and love.

Dementia may take much away; our friend may not even remember the story of the friendship we have shared. But we remember. We remember the things our friend loves, the things that bring our friend joy. Our conversations with our friend will be different than they once were. But we can be with our friend in the present moment, sharing laughter, pleasure, joy and love. And if we can overcome our own anxiety and simply be in the moment with our friend, we will make the delightful discovery that we too will experience joy. In the end, the pleasure of genuine friendship lies not in the topics we discuss, but the connection we share with one another.

Precious God, who, in Jesus has named us friends, help us to be faithful in our friendships with one another. Particularly when our cherished friend journeys into memory loss or confusion, help us to overcome our discomfort and teach us how to be present to our friend in laughter, pleasure, joy and love. Amen.

Rev. John T. McFadden, MDiv (The United Church of Christ)

HE FINISHED HIS RACE

Read 2 Timothy 4:6-8

I have fought the good fight, I have finished the race, I have kept the faith.
- 2 Timothy 4:7

Drue, my brother-in-law, was the constant caregiver for my sister, Pat, who struggled with vascular dementia for several years. I could only be a distant help, offering support by phone and prayers on his behalf. Drue had retired from the United States Army as a Colonel, serving two terms with distinction in Vietnam. He served his country with utmost devotion, and brought that same devotion to caring for his wife.

As the task grew more demanding, and brought him to near exhaustion, somehow he maintained his loving care. Our family begged him to get help, but he refused, saying, "This is my duty." At times when I called, he seemed spent and weary, but kept his optimistic spirit, even telling me about humorous events as he took care of Pat. When she became confused and at times belligerent, he would respond with incredible kindness and understanding. His last full measure of devotion was to lay down his life for his wife.

When Pat died, Drue told me, "I accomplished my mission: caring for Pat. Life is empty without her. I am ready to 'belly up.'" He had "fought the good fight, kept the faith and finished his race." Drue defied the wisdom that caregivers should care for themselves. He poured out life like an offering, denying his own needs for his wife's comfort. He received no medals as he did for his military service. But he was my hero, and his medals were the thanksgiving of his family.

The picture of his sad and forlorn face when he placed Pat's ashes into the ocean still haunts me. A few months after Pat died, Drue had a massive stoke from which he never fully recovered. The 36-hour days and nights had taken their toll. In a short time Drue died, and told his daughter shortly before he died, "Death is part of life. No one lives forever." Whenever caregiving is mentioned, Drue's loving care for his wife will always come to mind. His last tour of duty became a gift to all of our family.

Although people who care for persons with dementia need respite, and a break, we cannot but fail to admire those who lose their lives in caring for a loved one. They leave a poignant memory of unconditional love.

Richard L. Morgan, PhD, Retired Clergy (Presbyterian Church, USA)

THE PRESENCE OF ABSENCE

Surely the Lord is in this place, and I did not know it. - Genesis 28:16

If I make my bed in Sheol, you are there. - Psalm 139:8

It has been years ago, but the visits to see Mother suffering from Parkinson's dementia are as real as yesterday. I was a distant caregiver, and lived miles away. Yet, each time I visited mother, I saw her progression downward, her descent into darkness, her death in slow motion. Mother once had a fantastic memory, and would entertain people with her stories. Soon her speech was gone and memory swept away like a quiet storm. When I visited her, I often wondered if she knew who I was, or even who she was. It was sad to see her mask-like face, trembling hands, and deafening silence. Her mind reminded me of an empty church, dark and deserted.

At my last visit before God's angels took her home, and her long journey into darkness ended, I sat in silence at her bedside, holding her hand, and looking for any sign of recognition. I had no words, but just a presence in her absence. Her favorite gospel hymn was "In the Sweet By and By," and I softly sang some of its lyrics to her:

"There's a land that is fairer than day, and by faith we can see it afar; for the Father waits over the way, to prepare us a dwelling place there. In the sweet by and by, we shall meet on that beautiful shore."

A glimmer of a smile appeared on her face, and I knew she heard.

Alzheimer's leaves a person physically present, but mentally absent. Yet, I learned that there is a presence in that absence. At first, I did not know that the Lord was in the darkness of her dementia, a Presence in her absence. Only later did I realize she was there, a living soul, and that even when God seems far away and unavailable, God is there, shrouded in darkness, but keeping watch over our lives with unending love. Indeed, one day, her darkness became brilliant light, "in a land that is fairer than day," and one day we shall meet on that beautiful shore.

Gracious God, teach us to know that when dementia robs people of their minds, their souls are still present, even as You are there when You seem distant and far away. Amen.

Richard L. Morgan, PhD, Retired Clergy (Presbyterian Church, USA)

AFTER DARKNESS: DISCOVERING LIFE'S BEAUTY

"The most beautiful people we have known are those who have known defeat, known suffering, known struggle, known loss, and have found their way out of the depths. These persons have an appreciation, a sensitivity, and an understanding of life that fills them with compassion, gentleness, and a deep loving concern. Beautiful people do not just happen." - Elisabeth Kübler-Ross, Death: The Final Stage of Growth, 1975

A loved one melts away at the hand of Alzheimer's. Cruel. Unfair. Illogical. In the eyes of many, it's the darkest, most distressing, most dreadful way to exit this world. Sometimes, I envision it as a lifelike character. A foreboding creature, he is immense in size and cloaked in black from head to toe. No sign of compassion and certainly not an ounce of mercy. There's no match for this indomitable monster.

We watch, and we wait. We do the very best we can each step of the way until one day everything stops. It's suddenly over, and we're left feeling lost and alone; so much of our identity wrapped up in caring for and loving the person who lived with Alzheimer's. There are moments when we feel we can't go on. Or we don't want to.

It was a journey that changed us forever. We might characterize the road traveled as treacherous, but what a gross understatement that would be. Never again will we be the same as we once were. Any hint of innocence is gone after watching the destruction of Alzheimer's, but in an odd way and without hesitation, many of us can say we're better human beings for having lived through it.

Those of us left behind have known the ultimate defeat. We've seen senseless suffering, and we've lost so much. But at the end of the day, we survived. We're stronger, more compassionate, and have a better sense of what's truly important. We realize that tomorrow isn't promised and we begin to notice the abundance of God's precious gifts before us.

Suddenly, a vibrant patch of wildflowers becomes one of the most beautiful sights in the world. We recognize and appreciate little things: the aroma of freshly-brewed coffee filling the house before the sun comes up or the friendly person who smiles and says hello in the elevator. We look up and realize the patterns the clouds form in the sky are a masterpiece and we taste a sweet, juicy August peach in a way we never have before.

We look at life through a different lens, and perhaps through this journey, we even find the life purpose for which we've always yearned.

Heavenly Father, thank you for giving me another day on this Earth. In my darkest moments, when I begin to question everything and feel like I'm drowning in sadness, please give me strength. Remind me that after darkness, light will come. Help me to see the abundant blessings in my path, and guide me in using my experience to lighten the load of others. Amen.

Ann Napoletan (Interdenominational)

COMFORT FOR THOSE LEFT BEHIND

When you go through deep waters I will be with you. When you go through rivers of difficulty, you will not drown. When you walk through the fire of oppression, you will not be burned up; the flames will not consume you. - Isaiah 43:2 (NLT)

I love the Lord because he hears my voice and my prayer for mercy. Because he bends down to listen, I will pray as long as I have breath! Death wrapped its ropes around me; the terrors of the grave overtook me. I saw only trouble and sorrow. Then I called on the name of the Lord: "Please, Lord, save me!" How kind the Lord is! How good he is! So merciful, this God of ours! The Lord protects those of childlike faith; I was facing death, and he saved me. Let my soul be at rest again, for the Lord has been good to me. He has saved me from death, my eyes from tears, my feet from stumbling. And so I walk in the Lord's presence as I live here on earth! - Psalm 116:1-4, 6-9a (NLT)

In the days and months following the end of my mom's eight-year journey with dementia, I found myself operating on autopilot. My car seemed to have a will of its own. I found myself turning into the nursing home parking lot, even though Mama had been in Heaven for three months. Sitting in my usual parking space, my heart was broken that I no longer had my "to do" list for Mom. My car was no longer loaded down with laundry, bath wash, socks, candy and elastic band bracelets and necklaces in vibrant colors. I no longer spent hours shopping for soft, flowing outfits that would resist food and urine stains.

You see, mourning and death is an individual journey. In the four days leading to my mom's death, I must have read Psalm 116 hundreds of times to her. Each time, she responded with softened breaths. She had shared with me, prior to her coma, that she had prayed to the Lord to send someone to bring her home to Glory. She advised me that my dad had been to visit more often (he had been dead for several years). She often complained that he came to visit around meal time and consumed her supper!

Dementia may have taken my mom, but this disease never stole her spirit. She remained faithful. I held her in my arms as she died. When she died, three words were released from her mouth. These three words were, "I love you." Remarkable, you see, as she had not been able to speak for three months prior to her death.

Each day, I wear a piece of her jewelry as a touch point of her. Today was a charm bracelet; tomorrow may be her silver cross earrings. But every day is a celebration of the gift she left behind: her love for me.

Dear Lord, when my heart breaks, I know that You hold my tears. You are my strength and my salvation. I celebrate my loved ones crossing into Your arms and ask for Your comfort during my moments of grief and doubt. Amen.

Laura Pannell, PhD, CPG (United Methodist)

WHOLE AND BEAUTIFUL,
JUST AS GOD CREATED IT TO BE

"There is in all visible things...a hidden wholeness."- Thomas Merton

When someone is diagnosed with dementia, we hear about plaques and tangles, brain physiology and how it is changing, losses and limitations, and how to manage behaviors. We are told that our mother, father, husband, wife, sister, brother, grandmother, grandfather, uncle, aunt, friend, is declining into a disease that robs us of everything that we once knew.

This is how my journey began as well. But something in this message did not make sense to me. I could not connect this information with the life of the precious person that I knew so well, and that was because I knew my mother's life to be more than the physiology of her brain, her intellect, talents and gifts, her personality and accomplishments.

I knew my mother's life to be sacred, and therefore when she was diagnosed my response was based on my faith, the one that she was so integral in teaching me...and this faith is grounded in the teachings of Jesus and all of the wisdom traditions. ALL life is sacred. We are to live our life with compassion. The greatest power in existence is the power of love.

It was therefore from this foundation that my experience with my mother was based. I also knew that if I believed what is eternal about life is our spirit then, "Mom is okay; she is whole and beautiful just as God created her to be." And this is what I found. My mother's strength and spirit continued to shine light on each person with whom she came in contact.

Because dementia has been known as the "long goodbye," our focus can be on the slow decline of our loved one. When we focus on limitations and losses, we are distracted from the beauty of life lived in the present moment. The spirit of life continues toward growth and awareness and remains whole and beautiful, just as God created it to be.

Gracious God, help us to see the beauty of life lived in the present moment. Amen.

Rev. Linn Possell (The United Church of Christ)

PAPA'S CHRISTMAS APPLES

Read Matthew 25:31-46

The King will reply, 'Truly I tell you, whatever you did for one of the least of these brothers and sisters of mine, you did for me." - Matthew 25:40 (NIV)

I have many poignant memories of my father, both before and after the diagnosis of Alzheimer's disease. None is more powerful and lasting than this one, about which I wrote a meditation for our church a few years ago:

> I can see my father's face clearly now, beaming with anticipation and glee as I snatched the stocking from the mantle. For he knew that nestled in the toe lay the fattest, juiciest, reddest, shiniest Christmas apples to be found. You see, it wasn't my obvious delight upon beholding a new bike or GI Joe doll that thrilled Papa most. Rather, it was the pulling out of the prize apples that gave the greatest satisfaction. Though I never saw the search, I know it was with loving care he must have chosen the fruit, polished the skin, and placed it in its familiar spot for tiny hands to grasp on Christmas morn. Memories such as these fill my life with rich aromas of Christmases past.
>
> Then came Christmas anew. The apples had been discovered. The Johnny West doll set upon his horse. The ambrosia served. The blessing begun.
>
> When came a knock; hesitant, but hopeful.
>
> Papa answered, and there he stood: reddened care-worn eyes, furrowed brown brow, curly white beard, tattered cap, shredded overcoat missing buttons, shoes with half soles. "Christmas Gift," he muttered, in hopeful resignation. With compassionate countenance, Papa turned to…the apples.
>
> Gathering up the finest fruit (the Christmas apples, oranges, bananas), he filled the old man's sack to overflowing. If Christmas came to the old man that day, it came in double portion to me.

Looking back through years and "spirit" eyes, I see myself in tattered clothes at Papa's back door seeking Christmas. The Son's finest fruit I don't deserve, but such I receive. You see, Papa's Christmas apples were polished for you and for me, and the stockings are always hung on Christmas morn.

God, call to mind rich memories, special times of meaning and relationship which can help to sustain us on particularly challenging days. Amen.

Daniel C. Potts, MD, FAAN, Elder (Presbyterian Church, USA)

LOST MEMORIES

By the rivers of Babylon we sat and wept when we remembered Zion. There on the poplars we hung our harps, for there our captors asked us for songs, our tormentors demanded songs of joy; they said, "Sing us one of the songs of Zion!" How can we sing the songs of the LORD while in a foreign land? If I forget you, Jerusalem, may my right hand forget its skill. May my tongue cling to the roof of my mouth if I do not remember you, if I do not consider Jerusalem my highest joy. - Psalm 137:1-6 (NIV)

Winter is a time in which the landscape seems so cold, barren, and dead. Spring and summer seem long gone, disappeared before our very eyes to be replaced by something else. Sooner or later in the progression of the disease, our loved ones or at least the ones we have known seem so foreign and far away to us. It is as though someone has come as a thief in the middle of the night and taken them from us, simply because they cannot remember. They cannot remember us, do not know how to speak, and cannot remember even who they are any longer. We now live in exile in a foreign land where we no longer know joy. We have reached the cold winter season of Alzheimer's.

Where is our joy? How can we be full of joy when we live in winter, a time of loss, scarcity, struggle, and grief? A strange landscape it is indeed. The lyricist of this ancient Biblical Song of Lament knew our experience. The writer of the lament is looking for something to hold onto in the harshness of his bitterness and suffering. The writer holds onto the only small thing he can: memories of happiness and glory gone by. Like a fleeting bloom, in the snows of winter the writer holds onto the memories of happier time.

But our loved ones cannot remember, so what is there to hold onto? Very little it seems, but it is enough. There is the fleeting sign that we are not merely a mind or body but a spiritual presence beyond our ability to remember. It is the ability to laugh, or cry, a small phrase our loved one can repeat in the middle of gibberish, or the verses of a hymn which the long-term memory can still locate somewhere in its recesses and the ability to sing or hum them out loud. Our loved one can still sing praises and still remember something, because even if the mind forgets, the soul remembers.

O Divine One, when the frost of winter comes into my life, help me to rest in the stillness of the experience. Also help me to see the telltale reminders of the summer passed and to regain hope for the spring and rebirth to come, when my loved one and I will experience new life. Amen.

Rev. Dr. William B. Randolph (United Methodist)

LOOK TO THE HILLS

I will lift up mine eyes unto the hills, from whence cometh my help. My help cometh from the Lord, which made heaven and earth. - Psalms 121:1-2 (KJV)

His troubled face told the story as he walked into the bedroom with fear in his eyes. "What's the matter?" I asked, as I rose to offer a comforting touch. He said nothing.

"What is it?" I continued. His steps were unsteady, and I urged him to sit on the bed.

"What is the matter?" I asked for the third time. With slowness of speech and pain in his voice, he said to me, "I can't remember *The Lord's Prayer!*"

"Sure you can," I replied softly.

"Do you want me to help you?" His head nodded, "Yes," but his uneasiness and shame were palpable. My heart hurt for him as I struggled to find a way to help this proud, beautiful retired pastor. How can I help him without making him feel like one of my elementary students? This was the man who had answered God's call on an Easter Sunday morning. This was the man who had entered college at age 42, graduated from seminary at age 57 and pastored in three states for 42 years. This was the man who began and ended every day in prayer and who lived a life committed to God's service. Yet on this day, having reached the age of 86 and being challenged with mild cognitive impairment, my beloved husband is panic stricken because he can't remember *The Lord's Prayer.*

"Our Father, who art in Heaven," I prayed and he repeated.

"Hallowed be Thy name," I led and he followed.

"Thy Kingdom come…" he said WITH me, and we prayed the rest of the prayer together. The look of relief that crossed his face reflected his internal battle with a condition he was afraid would get worse. The feeling of relief that entered my heart was a small victory in my struggle to preserve his dignity, to encourage his strengths, and to gracefully accept the reality of his condition.

This strong, independent man refused to succumb to the battle he fought daily. I struggled to find creative ways to keep him as active and as positive as possible. Two days before his death, he independently delivered Holy Communion to several shut-ins, and we thank God that he was able to finish his course with his head held high and his eyes toward Heaven. Together we looked to the hills for our help.

Dearest Father, thank you for lifting us up as we walk this mysterious journey together; for being our ever-present help; for teaching us to look to You. Amen.

Flores Green Reynolds (United Methodist)

THE VOICE IN A CAREGIVER'S HEART

My heart is sore pained within me: and the terrors of death are fallen upon me.
- Psalm 55:4 (KJV)

VOICE: My voice is often hushed by the rigors of survival. In my role as caregiver, I am overwhelmed with the mental exercise of trying to consider his feelings, ideas, and decisions even when they conflict with what I really want to do. I get depressed because there is so little time for me. Every action or inaction must be weighed on the scale of what is best for him. I think that perhaps this zeal to be selfless is my own invention. The guilt of dwelling on my pain makes me ashamed, yet I do love him.

Fearfulness and trembling are come upon me, and horror hath overwhelmed me.
- Psalm 55:5 (KJV)

VOICE: I see that he is no longer able to do some of the things he wants to do. His attempts frighten me, and I live in fear that he will injure himself, that his self-esteem will be damaged, that he will become physically ill from over-exertion, or that the realization of his inabilities will plunge him into a depression that I cannot fix. Sometimes this fear invades my dreams. Continuous fear is unsettling, yet I do love him.

And I said, "Oh that I had wings like a dove! For then would I fly away and be at rest."
- Psalm 55:6

VOICE: I try my best but am constantly overwhelmed with mental anguish. How can I hide this anguish from him when it hovers over us all the time? I comfort myself with food and fiction and TV and sports. My weight has soared, and my self-esteem has plummeted. I am often too tired to do what I need to do to get myself mentally and physically healthy, but I must try and maintain a strong, brave, positive persona. The demands of a job and other obligations coupled with mental anguish make me feel close to mental collapse. My pride makes that kind of collapse unacceptable, but sometimes I fear that it will happen anyway. Then what becomes of US? I must find my way, or WE will not make it. That is my dilemma, yet I do love him.

Cast thy burden upon the Lord, and he shall sustain thee.
- Psalm 55:22

VOICE: AMEN! Yet do I love him AND Him!

Holy Father, quiet the fear in my heart and comfort me with the words of our Savior, "I will never leave you nor forsake you." Amen.

Flores Green Reynolds (United Methodist)

MEANING

Then the word of the Lord came to him, saying, "What are you doing here, Elijah?" He answered, "I have been very zealous for the Lord... the Israelites have forsaken your covenant... and killed your prophets... I alone am left, and they are seeking my life..." He said, "Go... stand on the mountain... for the Lord is about to pass by." Now there was a great wind, so strong that it was splitting mountains... but the Lord was not in the wind; and... an earthquake, but the Lord was not in the earthquake; and... a fire, but the Lord was not in the fire; and... a sound of sheer silence. - 1 Kings:19:9b-12 (NIV)

Dag Hammarskjöld experienced, like caregivers, discouragement, depression, and despair. In 1952 he wrote, "What I ask for is unreasonable: that life shall have a meaning. What I strive for is impossible: that my life shall acquire a meaning. I dare not believe, I do not see how I shall ever be able to believe: that I am not alone."

How reminiscent that is of the feelings of many people caring for a person with dementia, and also of another man of God engaged in a life of action in the world: Elijah after his confrontation with the prophets of Baal (1 Kings:18). Hounded into the wilderness by an enraged Jezebel, Elijah cries, "I have been very zealous for the Lord, the God of hosts; for the Israelites have forsaken your covenant... I alone am left, and they are seeking my life, to take it away" (1 Kings 19:10). But God does not leave Elijah to suffer alone, inadequate to the task. The prophet is fed and ordered to "stand upon the mount before the Lord," whose might is displayed in wind, earthquake, and fire, but whose uplifting Presence is finally revealed instead in "a sound of sheer silence" (v.12). Elijah comes to realize, through this renewal of faith, that he is not alone and his life has meaning; thus he experiences a renewal of faith in himself to accomplish his work.

Hammarskjöld also experienced renewals in his life when facing "wilderness" situations, expressed in this moving comment on Whitsunday 1961: "I don't know Who—or what—put the question, I don't know when it was put. I don't even remember answering. But at some moment I did answer *Yes* to Someone—or Something—and from that hour I was certain that existence is meaningful and that, therefore, my life, in self-surrender, had a goal." Because of such experiences, Hammarskjöld was able to pray, "Before Thee in humility, with Thee in faith, in Thee in peace."

God, when we experience life's valleys, remind us that we have answered "Yes" to You. Restore in us a sense of Your abiding Presence, that we may know that life has meaning beyond earthly measure and that we are never alone. Amen.

The Reverend Stephen Sapp, PhD (Presbyterian Church, USA)

PRAYER

For thus said the Lord God, the Holy One of Israel: In returning and rest you shall be saved; in quietness and in trust shall be your strength. - Isaiah 30:15

Be still, and know that I am God. - Psalm 46:10

One thing that all deeply spiritual people have in common is a commitment to regular prayer and meditation, and not only as a time for *them* to talk to God but also as an occasion to let God speak to them. Dag Hammarskjöld was no exception in this regard, and surely in this lies one of the secrets of his spiritual strength. Among the earliest reflections recorded in his journal *Markings* is this keen insight: "How can you expect to keep your powers of hearing when you never want to listen? That God should have time for you, you seem to take as much for granted as that you cannot have time for Him."

How true that is. Don't all too many of us become so involved in all the activities and pressures of our 36-hour days when dealing with a person with dementia that it is all too easy to relegate God to, at best, a small slot on Sunday morning (if we're even that lucky)? And then we often feel that we don't get any guidance from God, or that we fail to receive the strength or support in a crisis that we desire from a real sense of God's presence. We feel let down, maybe even betrayed, by a God who has promised to be there in our times of need, but seems not to be.

Well, perhaps God *is* there, but we just can't hear God's voice because we feel we don't have the time (or energy!) to discern God's will or to recognize God's presence. We get so busy giving compassionate care to our loved one that we don't take the time to listen, to be still, to receive. Indeed, how *can* we expect to retain our powers of hearing when we never want to listen?

Maybe we need to take to heart those ancient words that God once spoke through the prophet Isaiah: "In returning and rest you shall be saved; in quietness and in trust shall be your strength" (30:15). Maybe we need to heed God's admonition through the Psalmist, "Be still, and know that I am God" (46:10).

Almighty God, no matter how busy we are, help us to be still for a few moments each day, not only to talk to You but, perhaps even more important, to listen to You. Grant us the wisdom to realize that we cannot possibly hear what You have to say to us if we are always talking and never willing to listen. Amen.

The Reverend Stephen Sapp, PhD (Presbyterian Church, USA)

SOMETHING BIGGER THAN ME

The LORD is my strength and my shield; in him my heart trusts. - Psalm 28:7

"Fading away," says Milton. "Fading away. Okay. Okay. Okay."

Part of the struggle with the confusion and aggravation of his dementia had resulted in Milton's becoming violent. There was an ugly scene and Milton had been committed to the state psychiatric hospital. But time, the progression of the disease and a change in medication has now left Milton calm and seemingly at peace. So today when I ask, "Milton, how are you?" he tells me that he is fading away but that is okay.

I look at Milton in his bed. He has closed his eyes and has a Mona Lisa half smile. Then I look over at Brenda, Milton's wife for 50 plus years, sitting in the plastic chair in the corner of the hospital room. Her mouth is tight, her face is pinched, and her eyes show fear and worry.

Milton is the one with the disease. Milton is the one who has gotten my attention. Of course I have asked Brenda how she is and gently told her to get some sleep, to eat enough to keep herself alive, and to check in with her primary care provider. But Milton is the one I come to see. And when I make my list of pastoral care visits, it is Milton's name I type in, not Brenda's. But now I see Brenda's tight face deeply shadowed in care.

Brenda looks surprised when I stand up and go to her. I lay my hands on her head and mark her forehead in the sign of the cross with the oil of anointing. She takes my hand and looks at me, she lets out a long slow breath, and her eyes glisten. "Thank you, Pastor. Thank you. There is Something bigger than me," she nods.

And I leave that room knowing that I as a clergyperson need to be keenly aware that caregivers also suffer. Caregivers need to be connected to their overarching faith tradition that is bigger than all of us combined.

God of grace and God of glory, thank you for being the strength of caregivers when they are weak. Keep clergy aware that they are the caregivers of the caregivers, we pray through Christ Jesus, Our Lord. Amen.

Pastor David M. Seymour (Evangelical Lutheran Church in America)

THE ROBE OF CHRIST

I will not leave you orphaned; I am coming to you. - John 14:18

"Pastor," says Phyllis, "you know that Karl was…a bit vain, I guess you could say. He always wanted to look like he just stepped off the cover of GQ, and most of the time he looked just like that, like some famous male model. That's one of the things that attracted me to him," Phyllis smiles, almost blushing.

"But as the Alzheimer's progressed," she goes on, "he lost all concern about his appearance. You saw him; you know what I'm talking about. That was not him; he would have been horrified at the way he looked. Anyway, at the funeral I was thinking about how attractive and how striking he had been. And then at the opening prayers the pall was placed over the coffin. And the worship book says that pall represents the robe of Christ."

"I've been thinking about that robe of Christ. You know, when a baby is baptized we give it the robe of Christ, but it's more of a little bib really. My point is that it doesn't fit very well. And then we wear that robe of Christ symbolically all of our lives. And you know, Pastor, that robe never fits any of us perfectly. Now Karl's clothes fit perfectly, but that robe of Christ that he wore…well, he had his shortcomings; we all do."

"But when I saw that pall placed over the coffin, it fit perfectly. And then, Pastor, you said—and I remember this perfectly; I don't remember your sermon, not a word of it, but I remember this perfectly—you said, 'In his baptism Karl was clothed with Christ. In the day of Christ's coming, he shall be clothed in glory.'"

Phyllis pauses and then speaks again, but this time her voice is softer. "That's what I remember about the funeral, that Our Lord is with us from cradle to grave…and always. I knew that all along, but to see it, to hear it, at the funeral…" Phyllis's voice trails off. She shakes her head and smiles as the tears softly begin to flow.

Thank you, Lord Christ, for Your promise that we will never be left alone, that You will be with us from the first until the last. Amen.

Pastor David M. Seymour (Evangelical Lutheran Church in America)

Evangelical Lutheran Worship (Minneapolis: Augsburg Fortress Press, 2006), p. 280

STRETCH OUT YOUR HANDS

Truly, I say to you, when you were young, you girded yourself and walked where you would; but when you are old, you will stretch out your hands, and another will gird you and carry you where you do not wish to go. - John 21:18 (KJV)

That's it, isn't it? That's the reason our stomach knots when we have a senior moment, misplace our car keys, forget an appointment. We are determined to stay healthy and fit and fiercely independent, to never grow old. But sometimes we feel the holy ground on which we stand shifting beneath our feet.

It happened to my husband Bob in his late fifties when he was diagnosed with "probable Alzheimer's disease." A UCC minister, faithful and optimistic by nature, he had spent a lifetime counseling others and reminding us that we are human beings, not doings. Nonetheless, at the beginning, he was immobilized by fears of what he would no longer be able to do and what he would become. But eventually, his long journey with Alzheimer's became Bob's greatest sermon. As his mind and body wasted, his spirit grew brighter. His face glowed when a loved one remembered his stories or sang familiar songs and hymns or held his hand. He appreciated the caregivers at his nursing home who dressed and bathed and fed and lifted him. His gentle and trusting nature asserted itself. He spoke very little in the last few years but the words he mumbled most were good...thank...love.

Hindsight

Looking back, you understand
he wasn't trying to ignore you or annoy,
he wanted to remember your answer
to the question he asked over and over again...

Looking back, you understand
the brawny fear he wrestled but couldn't name,
limping and alone in the dark,
and you are awed by the courage it took
to grab on to life as it slipped through his fingers.

You understand that friends and family pulled away
as if it were contagious, because they didn't know
what to do, what to say; didn't want to see
what dementia looked like.

What you can't understand, looking back,
is how his mind learned to accept its degradation
and his spirit, to the very end, could radiate with love.

God, You always remember us and hold us in the palms of Your hands. Amen.

Anne Simpson (The United Church of Christ)

CONTINUING TO GLORIFY GOD

Very truly, I tell you, when you were younger you used to fasten your own belt and go wherever you wished. But when you grow old, you will stretch out your hands, and someone else will fasten a belt and take you where you do not wish to go. (He said this to indicate the kind of death by which he, Peter, would glorify God.)
- John 21:18, 19

For those who have spent their lives actively serving God, the very idea of having to be the one served is abhorrent. Even more so is the possibility that they might lose the memory of God and all the blessings received throughout a lifetime.

For caregivers, dementia may even seem to be an experience of God's absence, a sense that God has abandoned their faithful loved one. In the above passage, Jesus anticipates a time when Peter can no longer actively serve him, when Peter cannot even take care of himself. Jesus reassures Peter that even in that extreme state of dependency (and perhaps forgetting who Jesus is) Peter will be able to—somehow—continue to glorify God.

Mary Ella, a resident of a dementia care facility couldn't remember what her name was. She became distressed and wailed to Jeannie, the aide who was helping her to dress, "What's my name—I can't remember who I am!" The aide, in deep grief and anger with God because her mother had recently been diagnosed with Alzheimer's disease, saw Mary Ella's anguish as her own mother's future, and her anger at God intensified. She told her patient that her name was Mary Ella. Upon being told, Mary Ella immediately calmed, smiled broadly, and responded with a chuckle, "Half the time I don't know who I am"— and then she pointed to the crucifix on her bedroom wall and said, "But He does, and that's all that matters!"

Jeannie claimed that Mary Ella's witness to the all-encompassing love of God, no matter what condition we are in, gave her back her faith. God enabled Mary Ella, in her dementia, to be a pure channel of God's grace for her caregiver.

Loving God, help us to trust that no matter what our—or our loved one's—physical or mental status, we will continue to serve and to glorify You, to be a pure conduit of Your grace—even if we aren't aware of doing so! (All the better for not being aware—no chance for us to take the credit!) Amen.

Jane Marie Thibault, PhD (Catholic/United Methodist)

PSALM 139 FOR CAREGIVERS

by Richard L. Morgan and Jane Marie Thibault (© 2008)

Oh God, you know my heart,

and only you understand how hard

I have tried to care for my loved one.

You know that I hardly have time to sit down

or care for myself;

you know the long hours I spend

working and serving my loved one.

Only you know the depth of anger I feel

toward my family for their lack of help

and you know the harsh words I often speak

to the one I love - even before I say them.

I find it hard to hear your gentle voice

telling me to slow down,

not to fall prey to anxiety,

and to stop and rest in you.

You bless me even when I fail miserably,

when I get down on myself,

when I feel guilty for not doing enough.

Such understanding and grace are

beyond my comprehension.

I can never get away from you;

I cannot outlive your love.

If I have good days with my loved one,

when they have flashes of recognition,

you are there, celebrating with me.

If I sink down into the pits of despair

when everything is going wrong,

you are also there.

If I allow my mind to wander to more pleasant places,

you are there.

When the darkness of being on call around the clock

engulfs me and I want to scream,

you stand beside me and calm me.

And when I am tempted to believe that

all of this effort is wasted,

when I think I am wasting my life,

caring for something that will never come to fruition,

you hold me closest to your heart.

You know what it is like to experience

dark nights of the soul

Even though my loved one has this dreadful

brain disease and no longer knows who I am,

I will still believe their soul is alive

and reaches out to me.

Even when they sit and stare into nothingness,

I know that you have knitted them in the womb

and made them a person,

and that nothing can ever take away their personhood.

Search me, O God, and know my heart.

This experience tests my faith,

but you will sustain me in my weariness;

You will help me get through this terrible time.

Help me to love my loved one with your love

and to hold their hands and stay with them

until they rest safely in your embrace.

From Jane Marie Thibault and Richard L. Morgan, *No Act of Love is Ever Wasted; The Spirituality of Caring for Persons with Dementia* (Upper Room Books, 2009).

ACKNOWLEDGEMENTS

Seasons of Caring would not have been possible without the vision, dedication, teamwork, warmth, patience and tireless devotion of our volunteer editorial team: Dr. Richard Morgan, Lynda Everman, Dr. Daniel Potts, Rabbi Steven Glazer and Max Wallack. Each has been deeply and personally affected by Alzheimer's or dementia. And each has devoted countless hours not only to this project but to bettering the lives of so many others affected by this disease. We are grateful also to the Potts family for allowing us to feature the watercolors of Lester Potts, Jr., providing a moment of reflection and beauty between seasons. USAgainstAlzheimer's and the ClergyAgainstAlzheimer's Network owe this gracious and generous group a debt of gratitude. Thank you to our esteemed contributors, who each helped realize this team's vision of an interfaith volume that would embrace Alzheimer's caregivers and their families and show people of faith united in their determination to bring Alzheimer's out of the shadows. We are grateful for your wisdom and belief that *Seasons of Caring* will make a difference.

Thank you also to designer Mindy Kim, who helped bring this volume to life and ensure that the look reflects the warmth and intelligence of the words on the page.

The ClergyAgainstAlzheimer's Network welcomes clergy, laity and faith organizations. It launched in July 2014 with the support of 110 founding members representing a wide spectrum of faith traditions from across the country, including Presbyterian, Baptist, Catholic, Lutheran, Jewish, Muslim, Methodist and Episcopalian, among others. As leaders of congregations and faith communities, our founders – like so many clergy and people of faith - are at the forefront of pastoral care for those with Alzheimer's, eldercare issues, hospice care and the dementia-friendly communities movement. We are grateful to our founders for your tireless work focusing the nation's attention on Alzheimer's and for passionately speaking out for the dignity of those who have Alzheimer's and dementia.

To our readers—we are continually inspired by the strength and generosity of the many caregivers whom we are fortunate to work with and know, and who courageously share their own Alzheimer's stories. And thank you to George and Trish Vradenburg, the founders of USAgainstAlzheimer's, for their unwavering support of *Seasons of Caring*, their encouragement of the entrepreneurial and collaborative spirit of our editorial team, and their belief that clergy and people of faith are a powerful and critical voice in our effort to stop Alzheimer's.

To learn more please visit www.SeasonsofCaring.org.

Virginia Biggar
Director, ClergyAgainstAlzheimer's Network

PERMISSIONS AND NOTES

The publisher gratefully acknowledges permission to reprint from the following copyright sources.

The poem "Downeaster" by Joseph Gombita, *Observations from the Writer's Chair: A Collection of Poems* (J&J Books, 2014). Used by permission of the author.

The poem "This is (to) Mary Margaret Yearwood" by James Fowler, *In Their Hearts: Inspirational Alzheimer's Stories* by Mary Margaret Yearwood (Victoria BC: Trafford Publishing Company, 2002): 147-148.

"Psalm 139 for Caregivers" by Jane Marie Thibault and Richard L. Morgan, *No Act of Love is Ever Wasted: The Spirituality of Caring For Persons with Dementia* (Upper Room Books, 2009). Used by permission of Upper Room Books.

CONTRIBUTORS

To learn more please visit www.SeasonsofCaring.org.

Rabbi Richard F. Address, DMin (p. 117)
Founder/Director, Jewish Sacred Aging
Mantua, NJ

The Reverend Dr. Jade C. Angelica, MDiv, DMin (p. 1, 35)
Author, *Where Two Worlds Touch: A Spiritual Journey Through Alzheimer's Disease*
Founder and Director, Healing Moments™ Alzheimer's Ministry
Spiritual Director
Dubuque, IA

Alan Arnette (p. 36)
Mountain Climber, Professional Speaker, Alzheimer's Advocate
Fort Collins, CO

Mobed Maneck Bhujwala (p. 37)
Chair, Greater Huntington Beach Interfaith Council
Huntington Beach, CA

The Reverend Richard Bresnahan (p. 38, 39)
Roman Catholic Priest
Moline, IL

Rita Bresnahan (p. 40)
Psychologist, Educator, Spiritual Director
Author, *Walking One Another Home: Moments of Grace and Possibility in the Midst of Alzheimer's* and *Listening to the Corn*
Seattle, WA

Richard Campbell, MEd (p. 69)
Co-author, *Writing Your Legacy - A Step-by-Step Guide to Crafting Your Life Story*
Stoney Creek, Ontario, Canada

The Reverend Brenda F. Carroll (p. 118)
Superintendent
Chattanooga District, Holston Conference of the United Methodist Church
Chattanooga, TN

The Reverend Donna B. Coffman, MDiv (p. 2, 70)
Founder, Caring Spirit
Fuquay-Varina, NC

Rabbi Susan S. Conforti (p. 3, 4, 119, 120)
Lead Chaplain, Hoag Hospital, Department of Pastoral Care
Newport Beach, CA

Gerald Cumer (p. 99)
Presbyterian Elder
Greensburg, PA

Deacon Michael Francis Curren (p. 121, 122)
Roman Catholic Deacon
Reading, MA

Deborah D. Danner, PhD (p. 100)
Assistant Professor, University of Kentucky, Sanders-Brown Center on Aging
Author, *The Alzheimer's Book for African American Churches, Granny Pearl's Toolkit*
(Video & Lesson Plan)
Lexington, KY

J. Norfleete Day, PhD (p. 41)
Associate Professor Emeritus, Beeson Divinity School
Birmingham, AL

Deacon Drew DeCrease (p. 5, 6, 71, 101)
Hospice Chaplain, Senior Independence
North Huntingdon, PA

Robin Dill (p. 123)
Author, *Walking with Grace: Tools for Implementing and Launching a
Congregational Respite Program*
Director of Grace Arbor, Congregational Respite Program of First United Methodist Church
Lawrenceville, GA

The Reverend Dr. Donovan Drake (p. 7)
Pastor and Head of Staff
Westminster Presbyterian
Nashville, TN

The Reverend Dr. S. Miram Dunson (p. 8)
Presbyterian Older Adult Ministries Network
Commerce, GA

The Reverend Dr. Charles Durham (p. 72)
Pastor and Head of Staff
First Presbyterian Church Tuscaloosa
Tuscaloosa, AL

The Reverend Paige Eaves (p. 73, 102)
Lead Pastor, University United Methodist Church
Irvine, CA

Ronna L. Edelstein (p. 124)
Part-Time Faculty, University of Pittsburgh English Department
Pittsburgh, PA

Lynda Everman (p. ii, 9, 103, 125)
Convener, ClergyAgainstAlzheimer's Network
Board Member, B.A.B.E.S. (Beating Alzheimer's by Embracing Science)
Irvine, CA

Pastor Bobby Fields, Jr. (p. 74, 75)
Pastor, Mt. Olive Baptist Church, Loudon, TN
Program Coordinator, Alzheimer's Tennessee, Inc., Knoxville, TN

The Reverend Catherine Fransson, MDiv (p. 126, 127)
Pastor of Spiritual Direction, Seattle First Baptist Church
Seattle, WA

The Reverend Dr. Michael Gemignani, PhD, JD (p. 42, 76, 128, 129)
Episcopal Priest
League City, TX

The Reverend Dr. Richard H. Gentzler, Jr., DMin (p. 104)
Adjunct Faculty, School of TransformAging, Lipscomb University;
United Methodist Clergy; Author, *Aging and Ministry in the 21st Century: An Inquiry Approach,*
and *Designing an Older Adult Ministry*. Co-Author, *Forty-Sixty: A Study for Mid-Life Adults,* and
Gen2Gen: Sharing Jesus Across the Generations
Gallatin, TN

Rabbi Steven M. Glazer, DHL, DD (hon) (p. 10, 43, 44)
Rabbi Emeritus, Congregation Beth Emeth, Herndon, VA
Principal, Glazer Consulting, Rockville, MD

Joseph J. Gombita (p. 105)
Author, *Observations from the Writer's Chair: A Collection of Poetry*
North Huntingdon, PA

The Reverend Barbara J. Hineline (p. 130)
Chaplain, Redstone Highlands
Greensburg, PA

Olivia Ames Hoblitzelle (p. 11, 45, 77, 131)
Author, *Ten Thousand Joys & Ten Thousand Sorrows: A Couple's Journey Through Alzheimer's*
Dharma Teacher, Therapist, Former Teaching Fellow, Mind/Body Medical Institute
Cambridge, MA

The Reverend Dr. James Howell (p. 12)
Sr. Pastor, Myers Park United Methodist Church
Charlotte, NC

The Reverend Darrick Jackson (p. 13)
Educator & Treasurer, Healing Moments™ Alzheimer's Ministry
Dean of Students, Meadville Lombard Theological School
Chicago, IL

The Rev. Phil Jamison, Jr. (p. 46)
Chaplain, Redstone Highlands Senior Living Community, No. Huntington, PA
Bereavement Coordinator, Samaritan Counseling Center, Sewickley, PA

Kirti Kaur Khalsa (p. 47, 48)
Sikh Dharma International Minister
Co-founder, Alzheimer's Research and Prevention Foundation
Tucson, AZ

Maria Khani, Educator (p. 106, 132)
Chair of the Women's Committee
The Islamic Institute of Orange County, Anaheim, CA
Senior Muslim Chaplain, Los Angeles Sheriff's Department

Rabbi Cary D. Kozberg, MAHL, DD, BCC (p. 14, 15, 49, 133)
Director of Spiritual Life, Wexner Heritage Village
Author, *Honoring Broken Tablets: A Jewish Response to Dementia*; Co-author, *Flourishing in the Later Years: Jewish Pastoral Insights on Senior Residential Care*
Columbus, OH

The Reverend James D. Ludwick (p. 16)
Hospice Chaplain, Otterbein Senior Living Community
Lebanon, OH

Jill T. Lutz (p. 50)
Irvine Stake Director of Interfaith Relations,
The Church of Jesus Christ of Latter-day Saints
Irvine, CA

The Reverend Asa Hendrickson Majors (p. 78)
Pastor, Bethel-Vonore United Methodist Churches
Vonore, TN

Marie Marley, PhD (p. 17, 79, 80, 134)
Professional Speaker and Author, *Come Back Early Today: A Memoir of Love, Alzheimer's and Joy* and numerous articles for the Huffington Post,
the Alzheimer's Reading Room and Maria Shriver's Architects of Change
Olathe, KS

Benjamin T. Mast, PhD (p. 18, 107)
Associate Professor & Vice Chair, Psychological & Brain Sciences;
Associate Clinical Professor, Family & Geriatric Medicine, University of Louisville
Author, *Second Forgetting: Remembering the Power of the Gospel During Alzheimer's Disease*
Louisville, KY

The Reverend Brian McCaffrey (p. 81)
Chaplain, LutheranCare, Clinton, NY
Chair, The Northeast Forum on Spirituality and Aging
Author of *Caring Connections* articles: *Naming Your Spiritual Journey: Recognizing the Dynamic Nature of Faith; Who Will I Be When I Die? Nurturing A Second Half of Life Spirituality*

The Reverend John T. McFadden, MDiv (p. 135)
Memory Care Chaplain
Co-author, *Aging Together: Dementia, Friendship, and Flourishing Communities*
Appleton, WI

The Reverend Hunter Mobley (p. 51, 82, 83)
Executive Pastor, Christ Church, Nashville
Nashville, TN